MW00990065

DRUGS 2004

LIPPINCOTT WILLIAMS & WILKINS
A **Wolters Kluwer** Company

Philadelphia • Baltimore • New York • London
Buenos Aires • Hong Kong • Sydney • Tokyo

Staff

Publisher
Judith A. Schilling McCann, RN, MSN

Editorial Director
William J. Kelly

Clinical Director
Joan M. Robinson, RN, MSN

Senior Art Director
Arlene Putterman

Art Director
Elaine Kasmer

Clinical Manager
Eileen Cassin Gallen, RN, BSN

Drug Information Editor
Melissa M. Devlin, PharmD

Editorial Project Manager
Elizabeth P. Lowe

Clinical Project Manager
Minh N. Luu, RN, BSN, JD

Editor
Patricia Nale

Clinical Editor
Lisa M. Bonsall, RN, MSN, CRNP

Copy Editors
Leslie Dworkin, Beth E. Pitcher, Trish Turkington

Digital Composition Services
Diane Paluba (manager), Donald Knauss (project manager), Joyce Rossi Biletz (senior desktop assistant)

Manufacturing
Patricia K. Dorshaw (manager), Beth Janae Orr (book production manager)

Editorial Assistants
Carol A. Caputo, Tara L. Carter-Bell, Arlene P. Claffee

Indexer
Deborah K. Tourtlotte

Visit our Web site at eDrugInfo.com

ISBN 1-58255-246-0
ISSN 1531-4308
MPRD04—D N O
06 05 04 03 10 9 8 7 6 5 4 3 2 1

Contents

How to use this book

Medical Pocket Reference: Drugs 2004 is designed to help you find essential drug information quickly. A list of all the abbreviations used in the drug entries appears first. Then the entries are organized alphabetically by generic name. Under each generic name you'll find common brand names. Canadian brand names are followed by an asterisk (*).

Each drug entry then shows the drug's pharmacologic class and (after the semicolon) the therapeutic class. Next is the pregnancy risk category and, where applicable, controlled substance schedule.

Pregnancy risk categories parallel those assigned by the Food and Drug Administration to reflect a drug's potential to cause birth defects.
● A: Adequate studies in pregnant women have failed to show a risk to the fetus.
● B: Animal studies haven't shown a risk to the fetus, but controlled studies haven't been conducted in pregnant women; or animal studies have shown an adverse effect on the fetus, but adequate studies in pregnant women haven't shown a fetal risk.
● C: Animal studies have shown an adverse effect on the fetus, but adequate studies haven't been conducted in humans. The benefits may be acceptable despite potential risks.
● D: The drug may pose risks to the human fetus, but potential benefits may be acceptable despite the risks.
● X: Studies in animals or humans show fetal abnormalities, or reports of adverse reactions indicate evidence of fetal risk. The risks involved clearly outweigh the potential benefits.
● NR: Not rated.

Drugs regulated under the Controlled Substances Act of 1970 are divided into the following schedules:
● I: High abuse potential, no accepted medical use
● II: High abuse potential, severe dependence liability
● III: Less abuse potential than schedule II drugs, moderate dependence liability
● IV: Less abuse potential than schedule III drugs, limited dependence liability
● V: Limited abuse potential.

Next is information about the drug's available forms—the drug's preparations and dosage strengths.

The last section of the drug entries covers major indications and the most common dosages ordered. In this section, the multiplication symbol (×) is used for the word *for* to save space. The following symbols indicate when dosage adjustments are needed for renally impaired (†), hepatically impaired(‡), immunocompromised (§), or debilitated patients (¶).

A new appendix lists look-alike and sound-alike drug names. Another appendix provides a list of drugs not affected by dialysis.

The index covers trade names and indications.

Guide to abbreviations

ABG	arterial blood gas	CrCl	creatinine clearance
ac	before meals	CSF	cerebrospinal fluid
ACE	angiotensin-converting enzyme	CSS	Controlled Substance Schedule
ADHD	attention-deficit hyperactivity disorder	CV	cardiovascular
AIDS	acquired immunodeficiency syndrome	CVA	cerebrovascular accident
		d	day
ALL	acute lymphocytic leukemia	dl	deciliter
ALT	alanine aminotransferase	DM	diabetes mellitus
am	morning	DVT	deep vein thrombosis
aPTT	activated partial thromboplastin time	D_5W	dextrose 5% in water
		ET	endotracheal
ASAP	as soon as possible	exam	examination
AST	aspartate aminotransferase	g	gram
bid	twice a day	GERD	gastroesophageal reflux disease
BM	bowel movement	GGT	gamma-glutyamyl transpeptidase
BP	blood pressure		
BPH	benign prostatic hyperplasia	GI	gastrointestinal
BUN	blood urea nitrogen	gram-neg	gram-negative
CA	cancer	gram-pos	gram-positive
CAD	coronary artery disease	gtt	drop
CBC	complete blood count	GU	genitourinary
chemo	chemotherapy	GYN	gynecologic
cm	centimeter	H	histamine
CMV	cytomegalovirus	HBV	hepatitis B virus
COPD	chronic obstructive pulmonary disease	Hct	hematocrit
		HDL	high-density lipoprotein

v

HF	heart failure	mcg	microgram
Hgb	hemoglobin	mEq	milliequivalent
HIV	human immunodeficiency virus	mg	milligram
HMG-CoA	3-hydroxy-3-methylglutaryl coenzyme A	MI	myocardial infarction
		min	minute
H_2O	water	ml	milliliter
hr	hour	mo	month
hs	at bedtime	MS	multiple sclerosis
HSV	herpes simplex virus	NaCl	sodium chloride
HTN	hypertension	ng	nanogram
IBS	irritable bowel syndrome	NG	nasogastric
IM	intramuscular	NSAID	nonsteroidal anti-inflammatory drug
INR	international normalized ratio	NSS	normal saline solution
intraop	intraoperative	OA	osteoarthritis
IOP	intraocular pressure	OCD	obsessive-compulsive disorder
IPPB	intermittent positive-pressure breathing	OM	otitis media
IU	international unit	oz	ounce
IV	intravenous	PAC	premature atrial contraction
kg	kilogram	PAT	paroxysmal atrial tachycardia
L	liter	pc	after meals
LDH	lactate dehydrogenase	PCN	penicillin
LDL	low-density lipoprotein	PE	pulmonary embolism
liq	liquid	periop	perioperative
m^2	square meter	PID	pelvic inflammatory disease
MAC	*Mycobacterium avium* complex	pm	evening
MAO	monoamine oxidase	PMDD	premenstrual dysphoric disorder
max	maximum	PO	by mouth

postop	postoperative	TB	tuberculosis
PR	by rectum	tbl	tablespoon
PRC	pregnancy risk category	TCA	tricyclic antidepressant
preop	preoperative	temp	temperature
prn	as needed	tid	three times a day
PSVT	paroxysmal supraventricular tachycardia	TSH	thyroid-stimulating hormone
PT	prothrombin time	tsp	teaspoon
PTT	partial thromboplastin time	UTI	urinary tract infection
PVC	premature ventricular contraction	VF	ventricular fibrillation
		VT	ventricular tachycardia
PVT	paroxysmal ventricular tachycardia	WBC	white blood cell
		WHO	World Health Organization
q	every	wk	week
qid	four times a day	wkly	weekly
RA	rheumatoid arthritis	wt	weight
RBC	red blood cell	yr	year
RDA	recommended dietary allowance		
RF	renal failure		
RNA	ribonucleic acid		
SC	subcutaneous		
sec	second		
SL	sublingual		
SSRI	selective serotonin reuptake inhibitor		
ST	sinus tachycardia		
staph	staphylococci		
strep	streptococci		
SVT	supraventricular tachycardia		

—

abacavir sulfate
Ziagen

Antiviral (antiretroviral); nucleoside analogue reverse transcriptase inhibitor
PRC: C

Available forms
Tablets: 300 mg; *Oral solution:* 20 mg/ml

Indications & dosages
➤ *HIV-1 infection*—**Adult:** 300 mg PO bid with other antiretrovirals. **Child 3 mo-16 yr:** 8 mg/kg PO bid; max 300 mg with other antiretrovirals.

acarbose
Precose

Alpha-glucosidase inhibitor; antidiabetic
PRC: B

Available forms
Tablets: 50, 100 mg

Indications & dosages
➤ *Type 2 DM, adjunct to insulin or metformin in type 2 DM*—**Adult:** 25 mg PO tid with main meal; adjust q 4-8 wk. Maintenance 50-100 mg PO tid. Max 50 mg tid in patients ≤ 60 kg or 100 mg tid in patients > 60 kg.

acebutolol hydrochloride
Sectral

Beta blocker; antihypertensive, antiarrhythmic
PRC: B

Available forms
Capsules: 200, 400 mg

Indications & dosages
➤ *HTN*—**Adult:** 400 mg PO daily in 1 dose or divided doses bid. Max 1,200 mg daily.†
➤ *Ventricular arrhythmias*—**Adult:** 400 mg PO daily divided bid; increase prn to 600-1,200 mg.†

acetaminophen (APAP, paracetamol)
Acephen, Aceta, Anacin (aspirin free), Apacet, Feverall, Genapap Children's, Neopap, Panadol, Tempra, Tylenol

Para-aminophenol derivative; nonopioid analgesic, antipyretic
PRC: B

Available forms
Caplets: 160, 500 mg; *Caplets (extended-release):* 650 mg; *Capsules:* 325, 500 mg; *Elixir:* 80 mg/5 ml, 120 mg/5 ml, 160 mg/5 ml; *Gelcaps:* 500 mg; *Liq:* 160 mg/5 ml, 500 mg/5 ml; *Oral liq:* 160 mg/5 ml, 500 mg/15 ml; *Oral solution:* 48, 100 mg/ml; *Sprinkle:* 80, 160 mg/capsule; *Suppository:* 80, 120, 125, 300, 325, 650 mg; *Tablets:* 160, 325, 500, 650 mg; *Tablets (chewable):* 80 mg

Indications & dosages
➤ *Pain, fever*—**Adult, child > 11 yr:** 325-650 mg PO q 4-6 hr prn; or 1 g PO tid or qid prn. Or, 2 extended-release capsules PO q 8 hr. Max 4 g daily. For long-term, max 2.6 g daily. **Child 11 yr:** 480 mg PO or PR q 4-6 hr prn. **Child 9-10 yr:** 400 mg

PO or PR q 4-6 hr prn. **Child 6-8 yr:**
320 mg PO or PR q 4-6 hr prn. **Child 4-
5 yr:** 240 mg PO or PR q 4-6 hr prn. **Child
2-3 yr:** 160 mg PO or PR q 4-6 hr prn.
Child 12-23 mo: 120 mg PO q 4-6 hr prn.
Child 4-11 mo: 80 mg PO q 4-6 hr. **Child
≤ 3 mo:** 40 mg PO q 4-6 hr prn.

acetazolamide
Acetazolam*, Dazamide, Diamox,
Diamox Sequels

acetazolamide sodium

*Carbonic anhydrase inhibitor; anti-
glaucoma drug, diuretic*
PRC: C

Available forms
Capsules (extended-release): 500 mg; *Injection:* 500 mg/vial; *Tablets:* 125, 250 mg

Indications & dosages
➤ *Glaucoma, preop treatment of acute
angle-closure glaucoma*—**Adult:** 250 mg
PO q 4 hr or 250 mg PO bid. *Extended-
release:* 500 mg PO daily or bid. To lower
IOP, 500 mg IV; then 125-250 mg IV q
4 hr.
➤ *Edema in HF*—**Adult:** 250-375 mg PO
or IV q am. **Child:** 5 mg/kg PO or IV q am.
➤ *Chronic open-angle glaucoma*—**Adult:**
250 mg-1 g PO daily in divided doses qid
or 500 mg (extended-release) PO bid.
Child: 8-30 mg/kg daily PO in 3 divided
doses.

acetylcysteine
Mucomyst, Mucosil-10, Mucosil-20

*Amino acid (L-cysteine) derivative;
mucolytic; antidote for acetaminophen
overdose*
PRC: B

Available forms
Solution: 10%, 20%

Indications & dosages
➤ *Thick mucus secretions*—**Adult, child:**
1-2 ml of 10% or 20% solution by direct
instillation into trachea up to q hr; or 1-
10 ml of 20% solution or 2-20 ml of 10%
solution by nebulizer q 2-6 hr prn.
➤ *Acetaminophen toxicity*—**Adult, child:**
140 mg/kg PO; then 70 mg/kg PO q 4 hr
× 17 doses.

activated charcoal
Actidose, Actidose-Aqua, CharcoAid,
CharcoAid 2000, CharcoCaps, Liqui-Char

*Adsorbent; antidote, antidiarrheal, anti-
flatulent*
PRC: C

Available forms
Capsules: 260 mg; *Oral suspension:* 12.5,
15, 25, 30, 50 g; *Powder:* 15, 30, 40, 50,
120, 240 g; *Tablets:* 250 mg

Indications & dosages
➤ *Flatulence, dyspepsia*—**Adult:** 600 mg-
5 g PO in 1 dose or 0.975-3.9 g PO tid pc.
➤ *Poisoning*—**Adult, child:** 1-2/kg (30-
100 g) PO or 10 times the amount of poison ingested, given as suspension in 120-

---

240 ml H$_2$O. Give within 30 min of ingestion of poison.

acyclovir sodium
Avirax*, Zovirax

Synthetic purine nucleoside; antiviral
PRC: B

Available forms
Capsules: 200 mg; *Injection:* 500 mg, 1-g/ vial; *Suspension:* 200 mg/5 ml; *Tablets:* 400, 800 mg

Indications & dosages
➤ *Mucocutaneous HSV infection in immunocompromised patients; genital herpes in immunocompetent patients—***Adult, child ≥ 12 yr:** 5 mg/kg IV q 8 hr × 7 d. **Child < 12 yr:** 250 mg/m^2 IV q 8 hr × 7 d.†
➤ *Initial genital herpes—***Adult:** 200 mg PO q 4 hr while awake (total 5 capsules daily); or 400 mg PO q 8 hr. Continue 7-10 d.†
➤ *Recurrent genital herpes—***Adult:** 400 mg PO bid ≤ 12 mo.†
➤ *Varicella infection in immunocompromised patients—***Adult, child ≥ 12 yr:** 10 mg/kg IV q 8 hr × 7 d. **Child < 12 yr:** 20 mg/kg IV q 8 hr × 7 d.†

adalimumab
Humira

Monoclonal antibody; antarthritic
PRC: B

Available forms
Injection: 40-mg/ml vial; *Prefilled syringe:* 40 mg/ml

Indications & dosages
➤ *Reduce signs and symptoms and inhibit progression of structural damage in patients with moderate to severe RA who haven't responded to disease-modifying antirheumatic drugs or methotrexate—***Adult:** 40 mg SC q other wk. Patients not taking methotrexate may benefit with 40 mg q wk.

adefovir dipivoxil
Hepsera

Acyclic nucleotide analogue; antiviral
PRC: C

Available forms
Tablets: 10 mg

Indications & dosages
➤ *Chronic hepatitis B—***Adult:** 10 mg PO daily.†

adenosine
Adenocard

Nucleoside; antiarrhythmic
PRC: C

Available forms
Injection: 3 mg/ml in 2-ml vials, 2-ml syringes, 5-ml syringes

Indications & dosages
➤ *PSVT—* **Adult:** 6 mg rapid IV push over 1-2 sec. If PSVT persists after 1-

2 min, 12 mg by rapid IV push; repeat 12-mg dose once prn.

albuterol (salbutamol)
Proventil, Ventolin

albuterol sulfate (salbutamol sulfate)
AccuNeb, Proventil, Proventil HFA, Proventil Repetabs, Ventolin, Ventolin HFA, Volmax

Adrenergic; bronchodilator
PRC: C

Available forms
albuterol *Aerosol inhalation:* 90 mcg/metered spray; **albuterol sulfate** *Tablets:* 2, 4 mg; *Tablets (extended-release):* 4, 8 mg; *Syrup:* 2 mg/5 ml; *Solution (for inhalation):* 0.083%, 0.5%

Indications & dosages
➤ *Bronchospasm*—**Adult, child ≥ 12 yr:** *Aerosol inhalant:* 1-2 inhalations q 4-6 hr. *Solution (for inhalation):* 2.5 mg tid or qid by nebulizer. *Tablets:* 2-4 mg PO tid or qid; max 8 mg qid. *Extended-release:* 4-8 mg PO q 12 hr; max 16 mg bid. **Child 6-12 yr:** 2 mg (1 tsp) PO tid or qid. **Child 2-6 yr:** 0.1 mg/kg PO tid up to 0.2 mg/kg tid; max 4 mg tid. **Adult > 65 yr:** 2 mg PO tid or qid.
➤ *Prevention of exercise-induced bronchospasm*—**Adult, child ≥ 4 yr:** 2 inhalations 15 min before exercise.

alendronate sodium
Fosamax

Osteoclast-mediated bone resorption inhibitor; antiosteoporotic
PRC: C

Available forms
Tablets: 5, 10, 35, 40, 70 mg

Indications & dosages
➤ *Osteoporosis in postmenopausal women; to increase bone mass in men with osteoporosis*—**Adult:** 10 mg PO daily or 70-mg tablet PO q wk with full glass of H_2O only, ≥ 30 min before 1st food, liq, or medication of day.
➤ *Prevention of osteoporosis in postmenopausal women*—**Adult:** 5 mg PO daily or 35-mg tablet PO q wk with full glass of H_2O only, ≥ 30 min before 1st food, liq, or medication of day.
➤ *Corticosteroid-induced osteoporosis*—**Adult:** 5 mg PO daily with full glass of H_2O only, ≥ 30 min before 1st food, liq, or medication of day. In postmenopausal women not receiving estrogen replacement therapy, 10 mg PO daily.
➤ *Paget's disease of bone*—**Adult:** 40 mg PO daily × 6 mo with full glass of H_2O only, ≥ 30 min before 1st food, liq, or medication of day.

allopurinol
Lopurin, Purinol*, Zyloprim

Xanthine oxidase inhibitor; antigout drug
PRC: C

Available forms
Powder for injection: 500 mg; *Tablets (scored):* 100, 300 mg

Indications & dosages
➤ *Gout*—**Adult:** Mild gout, 200-300 mg PO daily; severe gout, 400-600 mg PO daily. Divide doses > 300 mg. Same dosage for maintenance in secondary hyperuricemia. Max 800 mg/d.†
➤ *Hyperuricemia secondary to malignancies*—**Adult:** 200-400 mg/m²; max 600 mg/dl. **Child:** Starting dose 200 mg/m² IV daily. **Child < 6 yr:** 50 mg PO tid. **Child 6-10 yr:** 300 mg PO daily or divided tid.†
➤ *Prevention of gouty attacks*—**Adult:** 100 mg PO daily; increase wkly by 100 mg until serum uric acid ≤ 6 mg/dl. Max 800 mg PO daily.†

almotriptan
Axert

Serotonin-1 receptor agonist; anti-migraine drug
PRC: C

Available forms
Tablets: 6.25, 12.5 mg

Indications & dosages
➤ *Acute migraine with or without aura*—**Adult:** 6.25- or 12.5-mg tablet PO, with 1 additional dose after 2 hr if headache is unresolved or recurs. Max 2 doses/24 hr.‡

alosetron hydrochloride
Lotronex

Selective 5-HT₃ receptor antagonist; anti-irritable bowel drug
PRC: B

Available forms
Tablets: 1 mg

Indications & dosages
➤ *IBS in women who have had chronic symptoms for ≥ 6 mo, who have no GI tract abnormalities, and who don't respond to conventional therapy*—**Adult:** 1 mg PO daily. Increase dose to 1 mg bid, prn, after 4 wk. If adequate control isn't reached after 4 wk on bid therapy, discontinue drug.

alprazolam
Apo-Alpraz*, Novo-Alprazol*, Nu-Alpraz*, Xanax, Xanax XR

Benzodiazepine; anxiolytic
PRC: D; CSS: IV

Available forms
Oral solution: 0.5 mg/5 ml, 1 mg/ml (concentrate); *Tablets:* 0.25, 0.5, 1, 2 mg; *Tablets (extended-release):* 0.5, 1, 2, 3 mg

Indications & dosages
➤ *Anxiety*—**Adult:** 0.25-0.5 mg PO tid. Max 4 mg daily in divided doses. **Elderly or debilitated patients or those with advanced liver disease:** Initially 0.25 mg PO bid or tid. Max 4 mg daily in divided doses.
➤ *Panic disorders*—**Adult:** 0.5 mg PO tid; increase q 3-4 d in increments of 1 mg/d. Max 10 mg daily in divided doses. Or ini-

tially 0.5-1 mg PO (extended-release) daily; increase q 3-4 d in increments of 1 mg/d. Max 10 mg/d.

alteplase (tissue plasminogen activator, recombinant; t-PA)
Activase, Cathflo Activase

Enzyme; thrombolytic enzyme
PRC: C

Available forms
Injection: 50-, 100-mg vials; 2-ml vials for intracatheter instillation

Indications & dosages
➤ *Lysis of thrombi in acute MI*—**Adult ≥ 65 kg:** 100 mg IV over 3 hr as follows: 60 mg in 1st hr (6-10 mg given as bolus over 1st 1-2 min). Then 20 mg/hr × 2 hr. **Adult < 65 kg:** 1.25 mg/kg IV over 3 hr as described above.
➤ *PE*—**Adult:** 100 mg IV over 2 hr. Begin heparin at end of infusion when PTT or thrombin time returns to 2 times normal or less.
➤ *Acute ischemic stroke*—**Adult:** 0.9 mg/kg IV over 1 hr with 10% of total dose given as initial IV bolus over 1 min. Max 90 mg. *Note:* Give within 3 hr after symptoms and after intracranial bleeding is ruled out.
➤ *Restoration of function to central venous access device*— **Adult, child > 2 yr:** For patients > 30 kg, instill 2 mg in 2 ml sterile H_2O into catheter. For patients 10-30 kg, instill 110% of the catheter's internal lumen volume. Max 2 mg. After 30 min of dwell time, assess catheter function by

aspirating blood. If function is restored, aspirate and discard 4-5 ml of blood, then gently flush catheter with 0.9% NSS. If function isn't restored after 2 hr, repeat dose.

amantadine hydrochloride
Symadine, Symmetrel

Synthetic cyclic primary amine; antiviral, antiparkinsonian
PRC: C

Available forms
Capsules: 100 mg; *Syrup:* 50 mg/5 ml

Indications & dosages
➤ *Influenza type A virus*—**Adult ≤ 65 yr, child > 9 yr:** 200 mg PO daily in 1 dose or divided bid.† **Child 1-9 yr:** 4.4-8.8 mg/kg PO daily in 1 dose or divided bid, to 150 mg daily. **Adult > 65 yr:** 100 mg PO daily. Start ASAP after exposure, preferably 24-48 hr after symptoms appear. Continue × 24-48 hr after they disappear.†
➤ *Parkinson's disease*—**Adult:** 100 mg PO bid. For patients on other antiparkinsonians or seriously ill patients, 100 mg PO daily for 1-2 wk; then 100 mg PO bid. Max 400 mg/d.†

amifostine
Ethyol

Organic thiophosphate; cytoprotective drug
PRC: C

Available forms
Injection: 500 mg anhydrous base

Indications & dosages

➤ *Reduction of renal toxicity with repeated cisplatin administration in patients with advanced ovarian or non-small-cell lung CA*—**Adult:** 910 mg/m² daily as 15-min IV infusion, starting 30 min before chemo. If hypotension occurs and BP is abnormal within 5 min after treatment stops, use 740 mg/m² for subsequent cycles.

➤ *Xerostomia in patients having postop radiation for head or neck CA*—**Adult:** 200 mg/m² daily as 3-min IV infusion, starting 15-30 min before radiation.

amikacin sulfate
Amikin

Aminoglycoside; antibiotic
PRC: D

Available forms
Injection: 50, 250 mg/ml

Indications & dosages

➤ *Serious infection*—**Adult, child:** 15 mg/kg/d divided q 8-12 hr by IM or IV infusion. **Neonate:** Loading dose, 10 mg/kg IV; then 7.5 mg/kg q 12 hr.†

➤ *Uncomplicated UTI*—**Adult:** 250 mg IM or IV bid.†

amiloride hydrochloride
Midamor

Potassium-sparing diuretic; diuretic, antihypertensive
PRC: B

Available forms
Tablets: 5 mg

Indications & dosages

➤ *HTN; edema in HF*—**Adult:** 5 mg PO daily. Increase to 10 mg daily prn; max 20 mg daily.

aminophylline (theophylline ethylenediamine)
Phyllocontin, Truphylline

Xanthine derivative; bronchodilator
PRC: C

Available forms
Injection: 250 mg/10 ml; 500 mg/20 ml; *Oral liq:* 105 mg/ml; *Rectal suppository:* 250, 500 mg; *Tablets:* 100, 200 mg; *Tablets (extended-release):* 350 mg*

Indications & dosages

➤ *Bronchospasm*—**Patient not using theophylline:** Loading dose 6 mg/kg IV; then maintenance infusion. **Adult (non-smoker) not using theophylline:** 0.7 mg/kg/hr IV × 12 hr; then 0.5 mg/kg/hr. **Otherwise healthy adult smoker not using theophylline:** 1 mg/kg/hr IV × 12 hr; then 0.8 mg/kg/hr. **Child 9-16 yr not using theophylline:** 1 mg/kg/hr IV × 12 hr; then 0.8 mg/kg/hr. **Child 6 mo-9 yr not using theophylline:** 1.2 mg/kg/hr × 12 hr; then 1 mg/kg/hr. **Patient using theophylline:** Infusion of 0.63 mg/kg to increase plasma drug level by 1 mcg/ml. If no signs of toxicity, 3.1 mg/kg.

➤ *Chronic bronchial asthma*—**Adult, child:** 16 mg/kg or 400 mg (whichever is less) PO daily in divided doses q 6-8 hr (for rapidly absorbed forms). May increase by 25% q 2-3 d. Or, 12 mg/kg or 400 mg (whichever is less) PO daily in divided doses q 8-12 hr (extended-release). May increase by 2-3 mg/kg/d q 3 d.

amiodarone hydrochloride
Cordarone, Pacerone

Benzofuran derivative; antiarrhythmic
PRC: D

Available forms
Injection: 50 mg/ml; *Tablets:* 200, 400 mg

Indications & dosages
➤ *Recurrent VF, unstable VT*—**Adult:** Loading dose 800-1,600 mg PO daily × 1-3 wk until initial response; then 600-800 mg/d PO × 1 mo; maintenance 200-600 mg PO daily. Or, loading 150 mg IV over 10 min (15 mg/min); then 360 mg IV over next 6 hr (1 mg/min); then 540 mg IV over next 18 hr (0.5 mg/min). After 1st 24 hr, continue maintenance infusion of 720 mg/24 hr (0.5 mg/min).

amitriptyline hydrochloride
Apo-Amitriptyline*

TCA; antidepressant
PRC: D

Available forms
Injection: 10 mg/ml; *Tablets:* 10, 25, 50, 75, 100, 150 mg

Indications & dosages
➤ *Depression*—**Adult:** 50-100 mg PO hs; increase to 150 mg daily. Max 300 mg daily prn. Maintenance 50-100 mg/d PO or 20-30 mg IM qid. **Elderly, adolescent:** 10 mg PO tid and 20 mg hs daily.

amlodipine besylate
Norvasc

Dihydropyridine calcium channel blocker; antianginal, antihypertensive
PRC: C

Available forms
Tablets: 2.5, 5, 10 mg

Indications & dosages
➤ *Angina*—**Adult:** 5-10 mg PO daily.
➤ *HTN*—**Adult:** Initially 2.5-5 mg PO daily. **Elderly:** 2.5 mg PO daily. For small or frail patients, patients using other antihypertensives, or those with hepatic insufficiency, begin at 2.5 mg daily. Max 10 mg/d. Adjust over 7-14 d.

amoxicillin and clavulanate potassium
Augmentin, Augmentin ES-600, Augmentin XR, Clavulin*

Aminopenicillin, beta-lactamase inhibitor; antibiotic
PRC: B

Available forms
Oral suspension: 125, 200, 250, 400, 600 mg amoxicillin trihydrate and 31.25, 28.5, 62.5, 57, 42.9 mg clavulanic acid, respectively, per 5 ml (after reconstitution); *Tablets (chewable):* 125, 200, 250, 400 mg amoxicillin trihydrate and 31.25, 28.5, 62.5, 57 mg clavulanic acid, respectively; *Tablets (extended-release):* 1,000 mg amoxicillin trihydrate/62.5 mg clavulanic acid; *Tablets (film-coated):* 250, 500, 875 mg amoxicillin trihydrate and

125, 125, 125 mg clavulanic acid, respectively

Indications & dosages
➤ *UTI; lower respiratory infection, OM, sinusitis, skin and skin-structure infection, from gram-pos and gram-neg organisms*—**Adult, child ≥ 40 kg:** 250-500 mg PO q 8 hr. **Child < 40 kg:** 20-40 mg/kg PO daily in divided doses q 8 hr.

➤ *Acute OM with antibiotic exposure ≤ 3 mo, in child ≤ 2 yr or in daycare*—**Infant, child 3 mo-12 yr:** 90 mg/kg/d Augmentin ES-600 PO q 12 hr × 10 d.

➤ *Community-acquired pneumonia or acute bacterial sinusitis due to confirmed or suspected beta-lactamase producing pathogens and Streptococcus pneumoniae with reduced susceptibility to penicillin*—**Adult, child ≥ 16 yr:** 2,000 mg/125 mg (two extended-release tablets) q 12 hr × 7-10 d for pneumonia or 10 d for sinusitis.

amoxicillin trihydrate
Amoxil, Apo-Amoxi*, Novamoxin*, Nu-Amoxi*, Trimox

Aminopenicillin; antibiotic
PRC: B

Available forms
Capsules: 250, 500 mg; *Pediatric drops:* 50 mg/ml (after reconstitution); *Suspension:* 125 mg/5 ml, 200 mg/5 ml, 250 mg/5 ml, 400 mg/5 ml; *Tablets (chewable):* 200, 400 mg; *Tablets (film-coated):* 500, 875 mg

Indications & dosages
➤ *Systemic infection, UTI from gram-pos and gram-neg organisms*—**Adult, child ≥ 20 kg:** 250-500 mg PO q 8 hr. **Child < 20 kg:** 20 mg/kg PO daily in divided doses q 8 hr; in severe infection, 40 mg/kg PO daily in divided doses q 8 hr or 500 mg-1 g/m² PO in divided doses q 8 hr.

➤ *Uncomplicated gonorrhea*—**Adult, child > 45 kg:** 3 g PO with 1 g probenecid in 1 dose. Not for child < 2 yr.

➤ *Endocarditis prophylaxis for dental procedures*—**Adult:** 2 g PO in 1 dose 1 hr before procedure. **Child > 2 yr:** 50 mg/kg PO in 1 dose 1 hr before procedure.

➤ *Postexposure prophylaxis to PCN-susceptible anthrax*—**Adult, child ≥ 9 yr:** 500 mg/kg/d PO tid q 8 hr. **Child < 9 yr:** 80 mg/kg/d PO tid or in 3 divided doses for 60 d.

amphotericin B
Amphocin, Amphotericin B for Injection, Fungizone Intravenous

Polyene macrolide; antifungal
PRC: B

Available forms
Injection: 50-mg lyophilized cake

Indications & dosages
➤ *Fungal infection, meningitis*—**Adult:** Test dose of 1 mg in 20 ml D₅W infusion IV over 20-30 min. If tolerated, 0.25-0.3 mg/kg/d IV (0.1 mg/ml) over 2-6 hr. Increase gradually to max 1 mg/kg daily or 1.5 mg/kg q other d. If stopped for

≥ 1 wk, resume drug with initial dose and increase gradually.

amphotericin B cholesteryl sulfate complex
Amphotec

Polyene macrolide; antifungal
PRC: B

Available forms
Injection: 50 mg/20 ml, 100 mg/50 ml

Indications & dosages
➤ *Invasive aspergillosis in patient unable to take amphotericin B deoxycholate—***Adult, child:** 3-4 mg/kg/d IV at 1 mg/kg/hr. Give test dose before new course of treatment; infuse small amount (10 ml final preparation with 1.6-8.3 mg drug) over 15-30 min and monitor × next 30 min.

amphotericin B lipid complex
Abelcet

Polyene antibiotic; antifungal
PRC: B

Available forms
Suspension (for injection): 100 mg/20-ml vial

Indications & dosages
➤ *Invasive fungal infection in patient refractory to or intolerant of conventional amphotericin B treatment—***Adult, child:** 5 mg/kg daily IV at 2.5 mg/kg/hr.

amphotericin B liposomal
AmBisome

Polyene antibiotic; antifungal
PRC: B

Available forms
Injection: 50-mg vial

Indications & dosages
➤ *Fungal infection in febrile, neutropenic patient—***Adult, child:** 3 mg/kg IV infusion daily.
➤ *Systemic fungal infection in patient refractory to or intolerant of conventional amphotericin B treatment—***Adult, child:** 3-5 mg/kg IV infusion daily.
➤ *Visceral leishmaniasis in immunocompetent patient—***Adult, child:** 3 mg/kg IV infusion daily on d 1-5, 14, and 21. May repeat prn.
➤ *Visceral leishmaniasis in immunocompromised patient—***Adult, child:** 4 mg/kg IV infusion daily on d 1-5, 10, 17, 24, 31, and 38.
➤ *Cryptococcal meningitis in HIV patient—***Adult, child:** 6 mg/kg/d IV infusion over 2 hr. Infusion time may be reduced to 1 hr or increased prn.

ampicillin
Apo-Ampi*, Novo-Ampicillin*, Penbritin*

ampicillin sodium
Ampicin*, Penbritin*

ampicillin trihydrate
Principen

Aminopenicillin; antibiotic
PRC: B

Available forms

Capsules: 250, 500 mg; *Infusion:* 1, 2 g; *Parenteral:* 125, 250, 500 mg; 1, 2 g; *Suspension:* 125, 250 mg/5 ml (after reconstitution)

Indications & dosages

➤ *Systemic infection, UTI*—**Adult:** 250-500 mg PO q 6 hr. **Child:** 50-100 mg/kg PO daily, in divided doses q 6 hr; or 100-200 mg/kg IM or IV daily, in divided doses q 6-8 hr.†
➤ *Meningitis*—**Adult:** 8-14 g IV divided q 3-4 hr × 3 d; then IM if needed. **Child 2 mo-12 yr:** Up to 400 mg/kg IV daily × 3 d; then up to 300 mg/kg IM divided q 4 hr. May give with chloramphenicol, pending culture results.†
➤ *Uncomplicated gonorrhea*—**Adult:** 3.5 g PO with 1 g probenecid in 1 dose.†
➤ *Prophylaxis for* Salmonella *in HIV patient*—**Adult:** 50-100 mg PO qid × several mo.†
➤ *Prophylaxis for bacterial endocarditis before dental or minor respiratory procedures*—**Adult:** 2 g (IV or IM) 30 min before procedure. **Child:** 50 mg/kg IV or IM 30 min before procedure.

ampicillin sodium and sulbactam sodium
Unasyn

Aminopenicillin and beta-lactamase inhibitor combination; antibiotic
PRC: B

Available forms

Injection: 1.5, 3 g (1 or 2 g ampicillin sodium and 0.5 or 1 g sulbactam sodium, respectively)

Indications & dosages

➤ *Intra-abdominal, GYN, and skin-structure infection*—**Adult, child ≥ 40 kg:** 1.5-3 g IM or IV q 6 hr. Max 4 g sulbactam and 8 g ampicillin (12 g of combined drugs) daily. **Child ≥ 1 yr or ≤ 40 kg:** 300 mg/kg/d IV divided equally q 6 hr.†

amprenavir
Agenerase

HIV protease inhibitor, sulfonamide; antiretroviral
PRC: C

Available forms

Capsules: 50, 150 mg; *Oral solution:* 15 mg/ml

Indications & dosages

➤ *HIV-1 infection*—**Adult, child 13-16 yr ≥ 50 kg:** *Capsules:* 1,200 mg PO bid. *Oral solution:* 1,400 mg PO bid. **Child 13-16 yr < 50 kg, 4-12 yr:** *Capsules:* 20 mg/kg PO bid or 15 mg/kg PO tid (max 2,400 mg/d). *Oral solution:* 22.5 mg/kg PO (1.5 ml/kg) bid or 17 mg/kg PO (1.1 ml/kg) tid (max 2,800 mg/d). Give with other antiretroviral.‡

---

§ Adjust in immunocompromised patients   ¶Adjust in debilitated patients

anakinra
Kineret

Lymphokine immunoregulator; immunologic agent, antirheumatic
PRC: B

Available forms
Injection: 100 mg/ml in a prefilled glass syringe

Indications & dosages
➤ *Moderately to severely active RA after one or more disease-modifying antirheumatic drugs fails*—**Adult:** 100 mg SC daily.

argatroban
Argatroban

Direct thrombin inhibitor; anticoagulant
PRC: B

Available forms
Injection: 100 mg/ml

Indications & dosages
➤ *Prophylaxis or treatment of thrombosis in patient with heparin-induced thrombocytopenia (HIT)*—**Adult:** 2 mcg/kg/min, as a continuous IV infusion; adjust dose until steady-state aPTT is 1.5-3 times initial baseline value, not to exceed 100 sec; max dose, 10 mcg/kg/min.‡
➤ *Anticoagulation in patients with or at risk for HIT during percutaneous coronary interventions*—**Adult:** 350 mcg/kg IV bolus over 3 to 5 min; continuous IV infusion of 25 mcg/kg/min. Activated clotting time (ACT) should be checked 5-

10 min after bolus dose. If ACT < 300 sec, give bolus of 150 mcg/kg and increase infusion to 30 mcg/kg/min; if ACT > 450 sec, decrease infusion to 15 mcg/kg/min. Recheck ACT in 5-10 min. In case of dissection, impending abrupt closure, thrombus formation during procedure, or inability to achieve or maintain ACT > 300 sec, give additional bolus of 150 mcg/kg and increase infusion to 40 mcg/kg/min. Check ACT again after 5-10 min.‡

aripiprazole
Abilify

Psychotropic; atypical antipsychotic
PRC: C

Available forms
Tablets: 10, 15, 20, 30 mg

Indications & dosages
➤ *Schizophrenia*—**Adult:** 10 to 15 mg PO daily; increase to max daily dose of 30 mg prn after ≥ 2 wk. Adjust dose if given with CYP 3A4 or CYP 2D6 inhibitors or CYP 3A4 inducers.

aspirin (acetylsalicylic acid)
ASA, Ascriptin, Bayer Timed-Release, Bufferin, Ecotrin

Salicylate; nonopioid analgesic, antipyretic, anti-inflammatory, platelet aggregation inhibitor
PRC: D

Available forms
Chewing gum: 227.5 mg; *Suppository:* 120, 200, 300, 600 mg; *Tablets:* 325,

---

500 mg; *Tablets (chewable):* 81 mg; *Tablets (controlled-release):* 800 mg; *Tablets (delayed-release, enteric-coated):* 81, 162, 325, 500, 650, 975 mg; *Tablets (timed-release):* 650 mg

Indications & dosages
➤ *RA, other inflammatory conditions*— **Adult:** 2.4-3.6 g PO daily in divided doses. Maintenance 3.2-6 g PO daily in divided doses.
➤ *Pain, fever*—**Adult, child > 11 yr:** 325-650 mg PO or PR q 4 hr, prn. **Child 2-11 yr:** 10-15 mg/kg PO or PR q 4 hr; max 60-80 mg/kg/d.
➤ *MI prophylaxis*—**Adult:** 160-325 mg PO daily.

atenolol
Apo-Atenolol*, Nu-Atenol*, Tenormin

Beta blocker; antihypertensive, anti-anginal
PRC: D

Available forms
Injection: 5 mg/10 ml; *Tablets:* 25, 50, 100 mg

Indications & dosages
➤ *HTN*—**Adult:** 50 mg PO daily; increase to 100 mg daily after 7-14 d.†
➤ *Angina pectoris*—**Adult:** 50 mg PO daily; increase to 100 mg daily after 7 d. Max 200 mg daily.†
➤ *Acute MI*—**Adult:** 5 mg IV over 5 min; repeat 10 min later. After additional 10 min, 50 mg PO; then 50 mg PO in 12 hr. Then, 100 mg PO daily (or 50 mg bid) ≥ 7 d.†

atomoxetine hydrochloride
Strattera

SSRI; ADHD drug
PRC: C

Available forms
Capsules: 10, 18, 25, 40, 60 mg

Indications & dosages
➤ *ADHD*—**Adult, child > 70 kg:** 40 mg PO daily; increase after 3 days to target dose of 80 mg/d (as a single am dose, or 2 evenly divided doses in the morning and late afternoon or early evening). After 2-4 wk, increase to max of 100 mg/d prn. **Child ≤ 70 kg:** 0.5 mg/kg PO daily; increase after 3 d to target dose of 1.2 mg/kg/d (as a single am dose, or 2 evenly divided doses in the morning and late afternoon or early evening). Max 1.4 mg/kg or 100 mg daily, whichever is less.‡

atorvastatin calcium
Lipitor

HMG-CoA reductase inhibitor; antilipemic
PRC: X

Available forms
Tablets: 10, 20, 40, 80 mg

Indications & dosages
➤ *Primary hypercholesterolemia and mixed dyslipidemia*—**Adult:** 10-20 mg PO daily. Patients who require > 45% reduction in LDL cholesterol, start with 40 mg daily. Range, 10-80 mg daily.
➤ *Homozygous familial hypercholesterolemia*—**Adult:** 10-80 mg PO daily.

➤ *Heterozygous familial hypercholester-olemia*—**Child 10-17 yr:** 10 mg PO daily; max 20 mg/d. Adjust at intervals of ≥ 4 wk.

atropine sulfate (systemic)

Anticholinergic, belladonna alkaloid; anti-arrhythmic, vagolytic
PRC: C

Available forms

Injection: 0.05, 0.1, 0.3, 0.4, 0.5, 0.8, 1 mg/ml; *Tablets:* 0.4 mg

Indications & dosages

➤ *Symptomatic bradycardia, bradyar-rhythmia*—**Adult:** 0.5-1 mg IV push; repeat q 3-5 min to max of 2 mg prn. **Child:** 0.01 mg/kg IV; may repeat q 4-6 hr; max 0.4 mg or 0.3 mg/m².
➤ *Preop to diminish secretions and block cardiac vagal reflexes*—**Adult, child ≥ 20 kg:** 0.4-0.6 mg IM or SC 30-60 min before anesthesia. **Child < 20 kg:** 0.01 mg/kg IM or SC (max 0.4 mg) 30-60 min before anesthesia.

azithromycin
Zithromax

Azalide macrolide; antibiotic
PRC: B

Available forms

Injection: 500 mg; *Oral suspension:* 100, 200 mg/5 ml; *Single-dose powder for oral suspension:* 1 g; *Tablets:* 250, 500, 600 mg

Indications & dosages

➤ *Bacterial exacerbation of COPD, community-acquired pneumonia, pharyngitis, tonsillitis, uncomplicated skin and skin-structure infections*—**Adult, child ≥ 16 yr:** 500 mg PO × 1 dose on d 1; then 250 mg daily on d 2-5. Total dose, 1.5 g. Or, for COPD exacerbation, 500 mg PO daily × 3 d.
➤ *Community-acquired pneumonia*—**Child ≥ 6 mo:** 10 mg/kg PO (max 500 mg) in 1 dose; then 5 mg/kg (max 250 mg) on d 2-5.
➤ *Otitis media*—**Child ≥ 6 mo:** 30 mg/kg PO × 1 dose. Or, 10 mg/kg PO (max 500 mg) in 1 dose; then 5 mg/kg (max 250 mg) on d 2-5.
➤ *Nongonococcal urethritis or cervicitis from Chlamydia trachomatis*—**Adult, child ≥ 16 yr:** 1 g PO in 1 dose.
➤ *Prevention of disseminated MAC in advanced HIV*—**Adult:** 1,200 mg PO q wk.

aztreonam
Azactam

Monobactam; antibiotic
PRC: B

Available forms

Injection: 500-mg, 1-, 2-g vials

Indications & dosages

➤ *UTI; septicemia; lower respiratory tract, skin and skin-structure, intra-abdominal, surgical, and GYN infection from susceptible gram-neg aerobic organisms; respiratory infection from Haemophilus influenzae*—**Adult:** 500 mg-2 g IV or IM q 8-12 hr. Severe infection, 2 g q

6-8 hr; max 8 g daily. **Child 9 mo-15 yr:** 30 mg/kg IV q 6-8 hr; max 120 mg/kg/d.

baclofen
Lioresal, Lioresal Intrathecal

GABA analogue derivative; skeletal muscle relaxant
PRC: C

Available forms
Intrathecal injection: 50, 500, 2,000 mcg/ml; *Tablets:* 10, 20 mg

Indications & dosages
➤ *Spasticity in MS, spinal cord injury—***Adult:** 5 mg PO tid × 3 d; then 10 mg tid × 3 d, 15 mg tid × 3 d, 20 mg tid × 3 d. Increase prn to max 80 mg daily.
➤ *Severe spasticity—***Adult:** *Test:* 1 ml of 50-mcg/ml dilution into intrathecal space by barbotage over ≥ 1 min. If poor response, give 2nd test dose (75 mcg/1.5 ml) 24 hr after 1st. If poor response, give test dose (100 mcg/2 ml) 24 hr later. Patients unresponsive to final test dose shouldn't have implantable pump. Maintain double effective dose and give over 24 hr. If test dose efficacy maintains ≥ 12 hr, don't double dose. After 1st 24 hr, increase dose prn by 10-30% daily.

balsalazide disodium
Colazal

GI drug; anti-inflammatory
PRC: B

Available forms
Capsules: 750 mg

Indications & dosages
➤ *Ulcerative colitis—***Adult:** 2.25 g PO (three 750-mg capsules) tid for total of 6.75 g daily × 8 wk.

basiliximab
Simulect

Recombinant chimeric human-murine monoclonal antibody IgG$_{1K}$; immunosuppressant
PRC: B

Available forms
Injection: 20-mg single-dose vials

Indications & dosages
➤ *Prophylaxis of acute organ rejection in patients receiving renal transplant when used as part of immunosuppressive regimen—***Adult, child ≥ 35 kg:** 20 mg IV ≤ 2 hr before transplant and 20 mg IV 4 d after transplant. **Child < 35 kg:** 10 mg given IV ≤ 2 hr before transplant and 10 mg IV 4 d after transplant.

beclomethasone dipropionate (oral inhalant)
QVAR

Glucocorticoid; anti-inflammatory, anti-asthmatic
PRC: C

Available forms
Oral inhalation aerosol: 40, 80 mcg/metered spray

---

§ Adjust in immunocompromised patients   ¶ Adjust in debilitated patients

Indications & dosages
➤ *Asthma*—**Adult, child ≥ 12 yr:** 40-80 mcg bid or 40-160 mcg bid (with inhaled corticosteroids). Max 320 mcg bid. **Child 5-11 yr:** 40 mcg bid; max 80 mcg bid.

benazepril hydrochloride
Lotensin

ACE inhibitor; antihypertensive
PRC: C (D, 2nd and 3rd trimesters)

Available forms
Tablets: 5, 10, 20, 40 mg

Indications & dosages
➤ *HTN*—**Adult:** *In patient not taking diuretics,* 10 mg PO daily. Adjust to 20-40 mg daily in 1-2 doses. *In patient taking diuretics,* 5 mg PO daily.†

benztropine mesylate
Apo-Benztropine*, Cogentin,
PMS Benztropine*

Anticholinergic; antiparkinsonian
PRC: C

Available forms
Injection: 1 mg/ml in 2-ml ampule;
Tablets: 0.5, 1, 2 mg

Indications & dosages
➤ *Drug-induced extrapyramidal disorders (except tardive dyskinesia)*—**Adult:** 1-4 mg PO or IM daily or bid.
➤ *Dystonic reaction*—**Adult:** 1-2 mg IV or IM; then 1-2 mg PO bid.

➤ *Parkinsonism*—**Adult:** 0.5-6 mg PO or IM daily. Initial dose 0.5-1 mg; increase by 0.5 mg q 5-6 d. Max 6 mg daily.

bepridil hydrochloride
Vascor

Calcium channel blocker; antianginal
PRC: C

Available forms
Tablets: 200, 300 mg

Indications & dosages
➤ *Stable angina*—**Adult:** 200 mg PO daily. Adjust after 10 d prn to maintenance dose 300 mg/d. Max 400 mg daily.

betamethasone
Betnesol*, Celestone

betamethasone acetate and betamethasone sodium phosphate
Celestonye Soluspan

betamethasone sodium phosphate
Celestone Phosphate

Glucocorticoid; anti-inflammatory
PRC: C

Available forms
betamethasone *Syrup:* 600 mcg/5 ml; *Tablets:* 500, 600 mcg; *Tablets (effervescent):* 500 mcg*; **acetate and sodium phosphate** *Injection (suspension):* acetate 3 mg and sodium phosphate (equivalent to 3 mg base)/ml; **sodium phosphate** *In-*

---

*Canadian   † Adjust in renal impairment   ‡ Adjust in liver impairment

jection: 4 mg (equivalent to 3-mg base)/ml in 5 ml

Indications & dosages
➤ *Severe inflammation, immunosuppression*—**Adult:** 0.6-7.2 mg PO daily; or 0.5-9 mg IM, IV, or into joint or soft tissue daily; **sodium phosphate-acetate suspension** 6-12 mg injection into large joints or 1.5-6 mg injection into small joints. Give both injections q 1-2 wk prn. *Note:* Don't give sodium phosphate-acetate suspension mixture IV.

betamethasone dipropionate
Alphatrex, Diprolene, Diprolene AF, Diprosone, Maxivate

betamethasone valerate
Betatrex, Beta-Val, Betnovate*, Luxiq, Valisone

Topical glucocorticoid; anti-inflammatory
PRC: C

Available forms
dipropionate *Aerosol:* 0.1%; *Cream, lotion, ointment:* 0.05%; **valerate** *Cream:* 0.01%, 0.05%, 0.1%; *Foam:* 0.12%; *Lotion, ointment:* 0.1%

Indications & dosages
➤ *Dermatitis*—**Adult, child:** Clean area; apply cream, ointment, lotion, or aerosol sparingly. Give dipropionate daily or bid; give valerate daily to qid. Max 45 g/wk for Diprolene cream; 50 ml/wk for Diprolene lotion.

betaxolol hydrochloride (ophthalmic)
Betoptic, Betoptic S

Beta blocker; antiglaucoma drug
PRC: C

Available forms
Ophthalmic solution: 0.5%; *Ophthalmic suspension:* 0.25%

Indications & dosages
➤ *Chronic open-angle glaucoma, ocular HTN*—**Adult:** 1-2 gtt 0.5% solution or 0.25% suspension bid.

bimatoprost
Lumigan

Prostaglandin analogue; antiglaucoma drug, ocular antihypertensive
PRC: C

Available forms
Ophthalmic solution: 0.03%

Indications & dosages
➤ *Reduce IOP in patients with open-angle glaucoma or ocular HTN*—**Adult:** 1 gtt in affected eye q pm.

biperiden hydrochloride
Akineton

biperiden lactate
Akineton

Anticholinergic; antiparkinsonian
PRC: C

---

§ Adjust in immunocompromised patients   ¶ Adjust in debilitated patients

Available forms
hydrochloride *Tablets:* 2 mg; **lactate** *Injection:* 5 mg/ml in 1-ml ampule

Indications & dosages
➤ *Drug-induced extrapyramidal disorders*—**Adult:** 2 mg PO daily to tid. Usual dose, 2 mg daily, or 2 mg IM or IV q 30 min. Max 4 doses or 8 mg daily.
➤ *Parkinsonism*—**Adult:** 2 mg PO tid or qid. Max 16 mg/d.

---

bisacodyl
Bisac-Evac, Bisacodyl Uniserts, Correctol, Dulcolax, Feen-a-mint, Fleet Bisacodyl, Fleet Laxative

Diphenylmethane derivative; stimulant laxative
PRC: NR

Available forms
Suppository: 10 mg; *Tablets (enteric-coated):* 5 mg

Indications & dosages
➤ *Constipation, bowel preparation*—**Adult, child > 12 yr:** 10-15 mg PO in am or pm; max 30 mg PO or 10 mg PR for evacuation before exam or surgery. **Child 6-12 yr:** 5 mg PO or PR hs or am.

---

bismuth subsalicylate
Bismatrol, Pepto-Bismol, Pink Bismuth

Adsorbent; antidiarrheal
PRC: C

Available forms
Caplets: 262 mg; *Oral suspension:* 130, 262, 524 mg/15 ml; *Tablets (chewable):* 262 mg

Indications & dosages
➤ *Diarrhea*—**Adult:** 30 ml or 2 tablets PO. **Child 3-6 yr:** 5 ml or ⅓ tablet PO. **Child 6-9 yr:** 10 ml or ⅔ tablet PO. **Child 9-12 yr:** 15 ml or 1 tablet PO. *Note:* Give all doses q ½-1 hr; max 8 doses/24 hr.

---

bisoprolol fumarate
Zebeta

Beta blocker; antihypertensive
PRC: C

Available forms
Tablets: 5, 10 mg

Indications & dosages
➤ *HTN*—**Adult:** 5 mg PO daily. Increase to 10-20 mg PO daily prn. Max 20 mg daily.†,‡

---

bivalirudin
Angiomax

Direct thrombin inhibitor; anticoagulant
PRC: B

Available forms
Injection: 250-mg vial

Indications & dosages
➤ *Unstable angina in patient undergoing percutaneous transluminal coronary angioplasty (PTCA)*—**Adult:** 1 mg/kg IV bolus just before PTCA; then begin 4-hr IV

---

infusion at 2.5 mg/kg/hr. After the 1st 4-hr infusion, another IV infusion at 0.2 mg/kg/hr ≤ 20 hr may be given prn. Give with 300-325 mg aspirin.†

bosentan
Tracleer

Endothelin receptor antagonist; antihypertensive
PRC: X

Available forms
Tablets: 62.5, 125 mg

Indications & dosages
➤ *Improve WHO class III or IV symptoms of pulmonary arterial HTN*—**Adults:** 62.5 mg PO bid × 4 wk. Increase to maintenance dose of 125 mg PO bid. In patients who develop aminotransferase abnormalities, decrease or stop drug until levels return to normal.

bromocriptine mesylate
Parlodel

Dopamine receptor agonist, semisynthetic ergot alkaloid, dopaminergic agonist; antiparkinsonian, prolactin release inhibitor, growth hormone release inhibitor
PRC: B

Available forms
Capsules: 5 mg; *Tablets:* 2.5 mg

Indications & dosages
➤ *Amenorrhea, galactorrhea, female infertility*—**Adult:** 0.5-2.5 mg PO daily; increase by 2.5 mg daily at 3-7 d intervals prn. Therapeutic dose, 2.5-15 mg/d.
➤ *Parkinson's disease*—**Adult:** 1.25 mg PO bid with meal; increase q 14-28 d. Max 100 mg daily prn.
➤ *Acromegaly*—**Adult:** 1.25-2.5 mg PO with snack hs × 3 d. Increase by 1.25-2.5 mg q 3-7 d prn. Max 100 mg/d.

budesonide
Entocort EC

Glucocorticosteroid; anti-inflammatory
PRC: C

Available forms
Capsules: 3 mg

Indications & dosages
➤ *Mild-to-moderate active Crohn's disease of the ileum or ascending colon*—**Adult:** 9 mg PO once daily in am × ≤ 8 wk. For recurrent episodes of active Crohn's disease, a repeat 8-wk course may be given.‡ May taper to 6 mg PO daily × 2 wk before complete cessation.

budesonide (nasal)
Rhinocort Aqua

Corticosteroid; anti-inflammatory
PRC: C

Available forms
Nasal spray: 32 mcg/metered spray (7-g canister)

---

§ Adjust in immunocompromised patients   ¶ Adjust in debilitated patients

Indications & dosages
➤ *Allergic rhinitis*—**Adult, child ≥ 6 yr:** 2 sprays in each nostril in am and pm, or 4 sprays in each nostril in am.

---

budesonide (oral inhalant)
Pulmicort Respules, Pulmicort Turbuhaler

Glucocorticosteroid; anti-inflammatory
PRC: B

Available forms
Dry powder inhalation: 200 mcg/dose; *Inhalation suspension:* 0.25 mg/2 ml, 0.5 mg/2 ml

Indications & dosages
➤ *Asthma*—**Adult previously using bronchodilators only:** 200-400 mcg inhalation bid; max 400 mcg bid. **Adult previously using inhalation corticosteroids:** 200-400 mcg inhalation bid; max 800 mcg bid. **Adult previously using PO corticosteroids:** 400-800 mcg inhalation bid; max 800 mcg bid. **Child ≥ 6 yr previously using bronchodilators only or inhalation corticosteroids:** 200 mcg inhalation bid; max 400 mcg bid. **Child ≥ 6 yr previously using PO corticosteroids:** Max 400 mcg bid. **Child 12 mo-8 yr** (Respules): 0.5-1 mg daily to bid via nebulizer.

---

bumetanide
Bumex

Loop diuretic; diuretic
PRC: C

Available forms
Injection: 0.25 mg/ml; *Tablets:* 0.5, 1, 2 mg

Indications & dosages
➤ *Edema*—**Adult:** 0.5-2 mg PO daily. May give 2nd or 3rd dose at 4-5 hr intervals prn. Max 10 mg/d. Or, 0.5-1 mg IV or IM. May give 2nd or 3rd dose at 2-3 hr intervals prn. Max 10 mg/d.

---

bupropion hydrochloride (antidepressant)
Wellbutrin, Wellbutrin SR

Aminoketone; antidepressant
PRC: B

Available forms
Tablets: 75, 100 mg; *Tablets (sustained-release):* 100, 150, 200 mg

Indications & dosages
➤ *Depression*—**Adult:** 100 mg PO bid × 3 d; then 100 mg PO tid prn. If no response after several wk, 150 mg tid. Max 450 mg/d. Or, 150 mg sustained-release tablet PO q am; increase to 150 mg PO bid as tolerated ≥ 4 d after 1st dose.

---

bupropion hydrochloride (nicotine replacement)
Zyban

Norepinephrine, serotonin, and dopamine inhibitor; nicotine replacement
PRC: B

Available forms
Tablets (sustained-release): 150 mg

Indications & dosages

➤ *Smoking cessation*—**Adult:** 150 mg PO daily × 3 d; max 300 mg PO daily in 2 divided doses ≥ 8 hr apart.

buspirone hydrochloride
BuSpar

Azaspirodecanedione derivative; anxiolytic
PRC: B

Available forms
Tablets: 5, 10, 15 mg

Indications & dosages

➤ *Anxiety*—**Adult:** 5 mg PO tid; increase q 3 d in 5-mg increments. Maintenance 20-30 mg PO daily in divided doses. Max 60 mg daily.

butorphanol tartrate
Stadol, Stadol NS

Opioid agonist-antagonist, opioid partial agonist; analgesic, adjunct to anesthesia
PRC: C; CSS: IV

Available forms
Injection: 1, 2 mg/ml; *Nasal spray:* 10 mg/ml

Indications & dosages

➤ *Pain*—**Adult:** 1-4 mg IM q 3-4 hr prn or around-the-clock; or 0.5-2 mg IV q 3-4 hr prn or around-the-clock. Max 4 mg/dose. Or, 1 mg nasal spray q 3-4 hr; repeat in 60-90 min prn.
➤ *Preop anesthesia or preanesthesia*—**Adult:** 2 mg IM 60-90 min preop.

calcitonin (salmon)
Miacalcin, Salmonine

Thyroid hormone; hypocalcemic
PRC: C

Available forms
Injection: 200 IU/ml, 2-ml ampule; *Nasal spray:* 200 IU/activation in 2-ml bottle

Indications & dosages

➤ *Paget's disease*—**Adult:** 100 IU daily SC or IM; maintenance 50 IU daily or 50-100 IU 3 times/wk.
➤ *Hypercalcemia*—**Adult:** 4 IU/kg q 12 hr IM. If poor response after 1-2 d, give 8 IU/kg IM q 12 hr. If poor response after ≥ 2 d, increase to max 8 IU/kg IM q 6 hr.
➤ *Osteoporosis*—**Adult:** 100 IU daily IM or SC. Or, 200 IU (1 spray) daily intranasally, alternating nostrils daily.

calcitriol (1,25-dihydroxycholecalciferol)
Calcijex, Rocaltrol

Vitamin D analogue; antihypocalcemic
PRC: A (D, doses > RDA)

Available forms
Capsules: 0.25, 0.5 mcg; *Injection:* 1, 2 mcg/ml; *Oral solution:* 1 mcg/ml

Indications & dosages

➤ *Hypocalcemia in long-term dialysis*—**Adult:** 0.25 mcg PO daily. Increase by 0.25 mcg daily q 4-8 wk. Maintenance 0.25 mcg every other d; max 1.25 mcg daily.

---

§ Adjust in immunocompromised patients   ¶ Adjust in debilitated patients

➤ *Hypoparathyroidism, pseudohypoparathyroidism*—**Adult, child > 6 yr:** 0.25 mcg PO daily. Increase at 2-4 wk intervals prn. Maintenance 0.5-2 mcg daily.

➤ *Hypoparathyroidism*—**Child 1-5 yr:** 0.25-0.75 mcg PO daily.

calcium carbonate
Alka-Mints, Calci-Chew, Chooz, Os-Cal 500, Tums 500

Calcium supplement; therapeutic agent for electrolyte balance
PRC: NR

Available forms
Contains 400 mg or 20 mEq elemental calcium/g. *Capsules:* 1,250 mg; *Gum:* 300, 450, 500 mg; *Oral suspension:* 1,250 mg/5 ml; *Powder packet:* 6.5 g (2,400 mg calcium)/packet; *Tablets:* 500, 600, 650, 667, 1,250, 1,500 mg; *Tablets (chewable):* 350, 420, 500, 750, 850, 1,000, 1,250 mg

Indications & dosages
➤ *Antacid*—**Adult:** 350 mg-1.5 g PO or 2 pieces of chewing gum 1 hr pc and hs prn.

➤ *Dietary supplement*—**Adult:** 500 mg-2 g PO bid-qid.

calcium polycarbophil
Equalactin, FiberCon, Fiber-Lax, FiberNorm, Mitrolan

Hydrophilic; bulk laxative, antidiarrheal
PRC: NR

Available forms
Tablets: 500 mg, 625 mg; *Tablets (chewable):* 625 mg

Indications & dosages
➤ *Constipation, diarrhea (acute IBS)*—**Adult, child ≥ 12 yr:** 1 g PO once daily-qid prn; max 4 g/24 hr. **Child 6-12 yr:** 500 mg PO once daily-tid prn; max 2 g/24 hr.

calcium salts
Calciject* (chloride), Calphron (acetate), Citracal (citrate), Neo-Calglucon (glubionate), PhosLo (acetate), Posture (phosphate)

Calcium supplement; therapeutic agent for electrolyte balance, cardiotonic
PRC: C

Available forms
acetate (253 mg or 12.7 mEq elemental calcium [elemental calcium]/g) *Injection:* 0.5 mEq Ca++/ml; *Tablets:* 667 mg; **chloride** (270 mg or 13.7 mEq elemental calcium/g) *Injection:* 10% solution in 10-ml ampule, vial, syringe; **citrate** (211 mg or 10.6 mEq elemental calcium/g) *Tablets:* 950 mg, 1.04 g; *Tablets (effervescent):* 2.376 g; **glubionate** (64 mg or 3.2 mEq elemental calcium/g) *Syrup:* 1.8 g/5 ml; **gluceptate** (82 mg or 4.1 mEq elemental calcium/g) *Injection:* 1.1g/5 ml in 5-ml ampule, 10-ml vial; **gluconate** (90 mg or 4.5 mEq elemental calcium/g) *Injection:* 10% solution in 10-ml ampule, 10-, 50-ml vials; *Tablets:* 500, 650 mg, 1 g; **lactate** (130 mg or 6.5 mEq elemental calcium/g) *Tablets:* 325, 650 mg; **phosphate, tribasic**

(400 mg or 20 mEq elemental calcium/g)
Tablets: 1,565 mg

Indications & dosages

➤ *Hypocalcemic emergency*—**Adult:** 7-14 mEq IV (as 10% gluconate solution, 2-10% chloride solution, or 22% gluceptate solution). **Child:** 1-7 mEq IV. **Infant:** Up to 1 mEq IV.
➤ *Hypocalcemic tetany*—**Adult:** 4.5-16 mEq IV. Repeat prn. **Child:** 0.5-0.7 mEq/kg IV tid or qid until controlled. **Neonate:** 2.4 mEq/kg IV daily in divided doses.
➤ *Cardiac arrest*—**Adult:** 0.027-0.054 mEq/kg chloride IV, 4.5-6.3 mEq gluceptate IV, or 2.3-3.7 mEq gluconate IV. **Child:** 0.27 mEq/kg IV. Repeat in 10 min prn; check serum calcium before giving further doses.
➤ *Magnesium intoxication*—**Adult:** 7 mEq IV. Subsequent doses prn.
➤ *Exchange transfusion*—**Adult:** 1.35 mEq IV with each 100 ml citrated blood. **Neonate:** 0.45 mEq IV after each 100 ml citrated blood.
➤ *Hyperphosphatemia*—**Adult:** 1,334-2,000 mg PO acetate tid with meals. Dialysis patient needs 3-4 tablets with meals.

candesartan cilexetil
Atacand

Selective angiotensin II receptor antagonist; antihypertensive
PRC: C (D, 2nd and 3rd trimesters)

Available forms
Tablets: 4, 8, 16, 32 mg

Indications & dosages

➤ *HTN*—**Adult:** 16 mg PO daily as monotherapy; range 8-32 mg PO daily in 1 dose or divided bid.

captopril
Apo-Capto*, Capoten, Novo-Captopril*

ACE inhibitor; antihypertensive, adjunctive treatment in HF
PRC: C (D, 2nd and 3rd trimesters)

Available forms
Tablets: 12.5, 25, 50, 100 mg

Indications & dosages

➤ *HTN*—**Adult:** 25 mg PO bid or tid. In 1-2 wk, increase to 50 mg bid or tid prn. If BP is uncontrolled after another 1-2 wk, add diuretic. If further BP reduction is needed, increase to 150 mg tid with diuretic. Max 450 mg daily.
➤ *HF, reduce HF after MI*—**Adult:** 6.25-12.5 mg PO tid. Increase to 50 mg tid prn. Max 450 mg daily.

carbamazepine
Apo-Carbamazepine*, Carbatrol, Epitol, Novo-Carbamaz*, Tegretol, Tegretol-XR, Teril

Iminostilbene derivative; anticonvulsant, analgesic
PRC: D

Available forms
Capsules (extended-release): 200, 300 mg; *Oral suspension:* 100 mg/5 ml; *Tablets:* 200 mg; *Tablets (chewable):* 100 mg;

Tablets (extended-release): 100, 200, 400 mg

Indications & dosages

➤ *Seizures*—**Adult, child > 12 yr:** 200 mg PO bid (tablet) or 1 tsp (suspension) PO qid. Increase wkly by 200 mg PO daily, in divided doses at 6-8 hr intervals prn. Max 1 g/d in child 12-15 yr or 1.2 g/d in child > 15 yr. **Child 6-12 yr:** 100 mg PO bid or ½ tsp suspension PO qid. Increase wkly by 100 mg PO daily. Max 1 g/d. **Child < 6 yr:** 10-20 mg/kg/d PO bid or tid (tablets) or qid (suspension). Max 35 mg/kg/d.

carbamide peroxide
Debrox

Urea hydrogen peroxide; ceruminolytic, topical antiseptic
PRC: NR

Available forms

Otic solution: 6.5% carbamide in glycerin or glycerin and propylene glycol

Indications & dosages

➤ *Impacted cerumen*—**Adult, child:** 5-10 gtt into ear canal bid × ≤ 4 d. Leave in ear canal 15-30 min; remove with warm H₂O.

carvedilol
Coreg

Beta blocker; vasodilator, antihypertensive
PRC: C

Available forms

Tablets: 3.125, 6.25, 12.5, 25 mg

Indications & dosages

➤ *HTN*—**Adult:** 6.25 mg PO bid. Get standing BP 1 hr after initial dose. If tolerated, continue dose × 7-14 d. Increase to 12.5 mg PO bid × 7-14 d prn, monitoring BP as noted. Max 25 mg PO bid. Reduce dose in patients with bradycardia (pulse rate < 55 beats/min).
➤ *HF*—**Adult:** 3.125 mg PO bid × 2 wk; if tolerated, increase to 6.25 mg PO bid. May double dose q 2 wk. Max for patients ≤ 85 kg, 25 mg PO bid; patients > 85 kg, 50 mg PO bid. Reduce dose in patients with bradycardia (pulse rate < 55 beats/min).
➤ *Left ventricular dysfunction post-MI*—**Adult:** Initially 6.25 mg PO bid × 3-10 d; then 12.5 mg bid up to 25 mg bid.

caspofungin acetate
Cancidas

Glucan synthesis inhibitor; antifungal
PRC: C

Available forms

Lyophilized powder for injection: 50-, 70-mg single-use vials

Indications & dosages

➤ *Invasive aspergillosis in patients refractory to or intolerant of other treatment*—**Adult:** Single 70-mg loading dose on d 1, followed by 50 mg daily thereafter. Give by slow IV infusion over about 1 hr. Duration of treatment based on severity of underlying disease, recovery from immunosuppression, and clinical response.†

---

cefaclor
Ceclor

2nd-generation cephalosporin; antibiotic
PRC: B

Available forms
Capsules: 250, 500 mg; *Oral suspension:* 125, 187, 250, 375 mg/5 ml; *Tablets (extended-release):* 375, 500 mg

Indications & dosages
➤ *UTI; respiratory, skin, soft-tissue infection; OM*—**Adult:** 250-500 mg PO q 8 hr. **Child:** 20 mg/kg daily PO in divided doses q 8 hr. More serious infection, 40 mg/kg daily; max 1 g daily. *Note:* For adult, child with pharyngitis or OM, may give daily dose in 2 equally divided doses q 12 hr.

cefadroxil monohydrate
Duricef

1st-generation cephalosporin; antibiotic
PRC: B

Available forms
Capsules: 500 mg; *Oral suspension:* 125, 250, 500 mg/5 ml; *Tablets:* 1 g

Indications & dosages
➤ *UTI; skin, soft-tissue infection; pharyngitis; tonsillitis*—**Adult:** 1-2 g PO daily, given daily or bid. **Child:** 30 mg/kg PO daily in 2 divided doses q 12 hr.†

cefazolin sodium
Ancef

1st-generation cephalosporin; antibiotic
PRC: B

Available forms
Infusion: 500 mg, 1 g/50-ml vial; *Injection (parenteral):* 500 mg, 1 g

Indications & dosages
➤ *Prophylaxis in contaminated surgery*—**Adult:** 1 g IM or IV 30-60 min preop; then 0.5-1 g IM or IV q 6-8 hr × 24 hr. For surgery > 2 hr, may give another 0.5-1 g IM intraop. Prophylaxis may continue × 3-5 g prn.†
➤ *Respiratory, biliary, GU, skin, soft-tissue, bone, joint infection; septicemia; endocarditis*—**Adult:** 250 mg IM or IV q 8 hr to 1.5 g PO q 6 hr. Max 12 g/d. **Infant > 1 mo:** 25-50 mg/kg or 1.25 g/m² daily IM or IV in 3 or 4 divided doses. May increase to 100 mg/kg/d.†

cefdinir
Omnicef

Broad-spectrum cephalosporin; antibiotic
PRC: B

Available forms
Capsules: 300 mg; *Suspension:* 125 mg/5 ml

Indications & dosages
➤ *Community-acquired pneumonia, exacerbation of chronic bronchitis, maxillary sinusitis, OM, uncomplicated skin and skin-structure infection*—**Adult, child**

---

§ Adjust in immunocompromised patients ¶ Adjust in debilitated patients

≥ **13 yr:** 300 mg PO q 12 hr or 600 mg PO q 24 hr × 10 d. (Use q-12-hr doses for pneumonia and skin infection.) **Child 6 mo-12 yr:** 7 mg/kg PO q 12 hr or 14 mg/kg PO q 24 hr × 10 d; max 600 mg daily. (Use q-12-hr doses for skin infection.)†
➤ *Pharyngitis, tonsillitis*—**Adult, child ≥ 13 yr:** 300 mg PO q 12 hr × 5-10 d or 600 mg PO q 24 hr × 10 d. **Child 6 mo-12 yr:** 7 mg/kg PO q 12 hr × 5-10 d or 14 mg/kg PO q 24 hr × 10 d.†

cefditoren pivoxil
Spectracef

Semisynthetic 3rd-generation cephalosporin; antibiotic
PRC: B

Available forms
Tablets: 200 mg

Indications & dosages
➤ *Acute bacterial exacerbation of chronic bronchitis from* Haemophilus influenzae, H. parainfluenzae, Streptococcus pneumoniae, Moraxella catarrhalis—**Adult, child ≥ 12 yr:** 400 mg PO bid with meals × 10 d.†
➤ *Pharyngitis or tonsillitis from* Streptococcus pyogenes—**Adult, child ≥ 12 yr:** 200 mg PO bid with meals × 10 d.†
➤ *Uncomplicated skin and skin-structure infection from* S. pyogenes—**Adult, child ≥ 12 yr:** 200 mg PO bid with meals × 10 d.†

cefepime hydrochloride
Maxipime

Semisynthetic cephalosporin; antibiotic
PRC: B

Available forms
Injection: 500 mg; 1, 2 g

Indications & dosages
➤ *UTI*—**Adult, child ≥ 12 yr:** 0.5-1 g (IM for *Escherichia coli* infection) or IV over 30 min q 12 hr × 7-10 d.†
➤ *UTI, pyelonephritis, skin infection, pneumonia, febrile neutropenic pediatric patients*—**Child 2 mo-16 yr ≤ 40 kg:** 50 mg/kg/dose IV over 30 min q 12 hr (q 8 hr in febrile neutropenia) × 7-10 d; max 2 g/dose.†
➤ *Severe UTI*—**Adult, child ≥ 12 yr:** 2 g IV over 30 min q 12 hr × 10 d.†
➤ *Pneumonia*—**Adult, child ≥ 12 yr:** 1-2 g IV over 30 min q 12 hr × 10 d.†

cefoperazone sodium
Cefobid

3rd-generation cephalosporin; antibiotic
PRC: B

Available forms
Injection: 1, 2 g

Indications & dosages
➤ *Respiratory, intra-abdominal, GYN, skin infection; bacteremia; septicemia*—**Adult:** 1-2 g q 12 hr IM or IV. Increase to 16 g/d in certain situations.‡

---

cefotaxime sodium
Claforan

3rd-generation cephalosporin; antibiotic
PRC: B

Available forms
Infusion: 1, 2 g; *Injection:* 500 mg; 1, 2 g

Indications & dosages
➤ *Periop prophylaxis in contaminated surgery*—**Adult, child ≥ 50 kg:** 1 g IM or IV 30-90 min preop. For C-section, 1 g IM or IV when umbilical cord is clamped; then 1 g IM or IV 6 and 12 hr later.†
➤ *UTI; lower respiratory tract, CNS, skin, bone, joint infection; GYN, intra-abdominal infection; bacteremia; septicemia*—**Adult:** 1 g IV or IM q 6-8 hr. Max 12 g daily. **Child 1 mo-12 yr or < 50 kg:** 50-180 mg/kg/d IM or IV in 4-6 divided doses. **Neonate ≤ 1 wk:** 50 mg/kg IV q 12 hr. **Neonate 1-4 wk:** 50 mg/kg IV q 8 hr.†

cefotetan disodium
Cefotan

2nd-generation cephalosporin, cephamycin; antibiotic
PRC: B

Available forms
Infusion: 1, 2 g piggyback; *Injection:* 1, 2 g

Indications & dosages
➤ *UTI; lower respiratory tract, GYN, skin, skin-structure, intra-abdominal, bone,*

joint infection—**Adult:** 1-2 g IV or IM q 12 hr × 5-10 d. Max 6 g/d.†
➤ *Periop prophylaxis*—**Adult:** 1-2 g IV × 1 dose 30-60 min preop. In C-section, give dose when umbilical cord is clamped.†

cefoxitin sodium
Mefoxin

2nd-generation cephalosporin, cephamycin; antibiotic
PRC: B

Available forms
Injection: 1, 2 g

Indications & dosages
➤ *Respiratory, GU tract, skin, soft-tissue, bone, joint, bloodstream, intra-abdominal infection; periop prophylaxis*—**Adult:** 1-2 g q 6-8 hr; max 12 g/d. **Child ≥ 3 mo:** 80-160 mg/kg/d in 4-6 equally divided doses; max 12 g/d.†
➤ *Surgery prophylaxis*—**Adult:** 2 g IM or IV 30-60 min preop; then 2 g IM or IV q 6 hr × 24 hr (72 hr after prosthetic arthroplasty). **Child ≥ 3 mo:** 30-40 mg/kg IM or IV 30-60 min preop; then 30-40 mg/kg q 6 hr × 24 hr (72 hr after prosthetic arthroplasty).†

cefpodoxime proxetil
Vantin

3rd-generation cephalosporin; antibiotic
PRC: B

---

§ Adjust in immunocompromised patients   ¶ Adjust in debilitated patients

Available forms
Oral suspension: 50, 100 mg/5 ml in 100-ml bottles; *Tablets (film-coated):* 100, 200 mg

Indications & dosages
➤ *Community-acquired pneumonia*—**Adult, child ≥ 13 yr:** 200 mg PO q 12 hr × 14 d.†
➤ *Exacerbation of chronic bronchitis*—**Adult, child ≥ 13 yr:** 200 mg PO q 12 hr × 10 d.†
➤ *Sinusitis from* Haemophilus influenzae, Streptococcus pneumoniae, *or* Moraxella catarrhalis—**Adult, child ≥ 12 yr:** 200 mg PO q 12 hr × 10 d. **Child 2 mo-11 yr:** 5 mg/kg PO q 12 hr × 10 d; max 200 mg/dose.†
➤ *UTI from* Escherichia coli, Klebsiella pneumoniae, Proteus mirabilis, *or* Staphylococcus saprophyticus—**Adult:** 100 mg PO q 12 hr × 7 d.†

---

cefprozil
Cefzil

2nd-generation cephalosporin; antibiotic
PRC: B

Available forms
Oral suspension: 125, 250 mg/5 ml; *Tablets:* 250, 500 mg

Indications & dosages
➤ *Pharyngitis, tonsillitis from* Staphylococcus pyogenes—**Adult, child ≥ 13 yr:** 500 mg PO daily × 10 d.†
➤ *OM from* Streptococcus pneumoniae, Haemophilus influenzae, *or* Moraxella

catarrhalis—**Infant, child 6 mo-12 yr:** 15 mg/kg PO q 12 hr × 10 d.†
➤ *Sinusitis*—**Adult, child ≥ 13 yr:** 250-500 mg PO q 12 hr × 10 d. **Child 6 mo-12 yr:** 7.5-15 mg/kg PO q 12 hr × 10 d.†

---

ceftazidime
Ceptaz, Fortaz, Tazicef, Tazidime

3rd-generation cephalosporin; antibiotic
PRC: B

Available forms
Injection (with arginine): 1, 2 g; *Injection (with sodium carbonate):* 500 mg; 1, 2 g

Indications & dosages
➤ *UTI; lower respiratory tract, GYN, intra-abdominal, CNS, skin infection; bacteremia; septicemia*—**Adult, child ≥ 12 yr:** 1 g IV or IM q 8-12 hr; max 6 g daily.† **Child 1 mo-12 yr:** 25-50 mg/kg IV q 8 hr (sodium carbonate prep).† **Neonate ≤ 4 wk:** 30 mg/kg IV q 12 hr (sodium carbonate prep).†

---

ceftibuten
Cedax

3rd-generation cephalosporin; antibiotic
PRC: B

Available forms
Capsules: 400 mg; *Oral suspension:* 90, 180 mg/5 ml

Indications & dosages
➤ *Exacerbation of chronic bronchitis*—**Adult, child ≥ 12 yr:** 400 mg PO daily ×

---

*Canadian   † Adjust in renal impairment   ‡ Adjust in liver impairment

10 d. Adjust dose in hemodialysis patients.†

➤ *Pharyngitis and tonsillitis from* Streptococcus pyogenes; *OM from* Haemophilus influenzae, Moraxella catarrhalis, *or* S. pyogenes—**Adult, child ≥ 12 yr:** 400 mg PO daily × 10 d. **Child < 12 yr:** 9 mg/kg PO daily × 10 d. **Child > 45 kg:** Max 400 mg PO daily × 10 d.†

ceftizoxime sodium
Cefizox

3rd-generation cephalosporin; antibiotic
PRC: B

Available forms
Injection: 500 mg; 1, 2 g

Indications & dosages
➤ *UTI; lower respiratory tract, GYN, intra-abdominal, bone, joint, skin infection; bacteremia; septicemia; meningitis*—**Adult:** 1-2 g IV or IM q 8-12 hr; max 2 g q 4 hr. **Child > 6 mo:** 33-50 mg/kg IV q 6-8 hr, up to 200 mg/kg/d in divided doses. Max 12 g/d.†

ceftriaxone sodium
Rocephin

3rd-generation cephalosporin; antibiotic
PRC: B

Available forms
Injection: 250, 500 mg; 1, 2 g

Indications & dosages
➤ *Infection*—**Adult:** 1-2 g IM or IV daily or bid.

➤ *Serious infection of lower respiratory and urinary tracts; GYN, bone, joint, intra-abdominal, skin infection; bacteremia; septicemia; Lyme disease*—**Adult, child > 12 yr:** 1-2 g IM or IV daily or in equally divided doses bid; max 4 g/d. **Child ≤ 12 yr:** 50-75 mg/kg IM or IV; max 2 g/d, in divided doses q 12 hr.

➤ *Meningitis*—**Adult, child:** 100 mg/kg IM or IV (max 4 g); then 100 mg/kg/d IM or IV given daily or in divided doses q 12 hr. Max 4 g/d × 7-14 d.

cefuroxime axetil
Ceftin

cefuroxime sodium
Zinacef

2nd-generation cephalosporin; antibiotic
PRC: B

Available forms
axetil *Suspension:* 125, 250 mg/5 ml; *Tablets:* 125, 250, 500 mg; **sodium** *Infusion:* 750 mg; 1.5 g premixed, frozen solution; *Injection:* 750 mg; 1.5 g

Indications & dosages
➤ *Serious infection; periop prophylaxis (injection); OM, pharyngitis; tonsillitis; UTI; lower respiratory tract, skin, skin-structure infection (PO)*—**Adult, child ≥ 12 yr:** 750 mg-1.5 g (sodium) IM or IV q 8 hr × 5-10 d; 1.5 g IM or IV q 6 hr in certain situations; bacterial meningitis, up to 3 g IV q 8 hr. Or, 250-500 mg (axetil) PO q 12 hr. **Child, infant > 3 mo:** 50-100 mg/kg/d (sodium) IM or IV in divided doses q 6-8 hr. Higher doses for meningi-

---

§ Adjust in immunocompromised patients   ¶ Adjust in debilitated patients

tis. Or, 125 mg (axetil) PO q 12 hr; bacterial meningitis, 200-240 mg/kg IV in divided doses q 6-8 hr.†
➤ *OM*—**Child < 2 yr:** 125 mg PO q 12 hr.
Child ≥ 2 yr: 250 mg PO q 12 hr.†
➤ *Early Lyme disease from* Borrelia burgdorferi—**Adult, child ≥ 13 yr:** 500 mg PO bid × 20 d.†
➤ *Sinusitis*—**Adult, child ≥ 13 yr:** 250 mg (tablet) PO bid × 10 d. **Child 3 mo-12 yr:** 30 mg/kg (suspension) PO daily in 2 divided doses × 10 d. Max suspension dose 1,000 mg/d; or 250 mg (tablet) PO bid × 10 d.

celecoxib
Celebrex

COX-2 inhibitor; NSAID
PRC: C

Available forms
Capsules: 100, 200 mg

Indications & dosages
➤ *Familial adenomatous polyposis*—
Adult: 400 mg PO bid with food ≤ 6 mo.‡
➤ *OA*—**Adult:** 200 mg PO daily in 1 dose or divided equally bid. In patients < 50 kg, start at lowest dose.‡
➤ *RA*—**Adult:** 100-200 mg PO bid. In patients < 50 kg, start at lowest dose.‡
➤ *Acute pain, primary dysmenorrhea*—
Adult: 400 mg PO initially; follow with 200-mg dose if needed on the 1st d. On subsequent d, 200 mg PO bid prn.

cephalexin hydrochloride
Keftab

cephalexin monohydrate
Apo-Cephalex*, Biocef, Keflex

1st-generation cephalosporin; antibiotic
PRC: B

Available forms
hydrochloride *Tablets:* 500 mg; **monohydrate** *Capsules:* 250, 500 mg; *Oral suspension:* 125, 250 mg/5 ml; *Tablets:* 250, 500 mg; 1 g

Indications & dosages
➤ *Respiratory, GI tract, skin, soft-tissue, bone, joint infection; OM from* Escherichia coli *and other coliform bacteria, group A beta-hemolytic strep,* Klebsiella, Proteus mirabilis, Streptococcus pneumoniae, *and staph*—**Adult:** 250 mg-1 g PO q 6 hr. **Child:** 6-12 mg/kg PO q 6 hr (monohydrate). Max 25 mg/kg q 6 hr.

cetirizine hydrochloride
Zyrtec

Selective H$_1$-receptor antagonist; antihistamine
PRC: B

Available forms
Oral solution: 5 mg/ml; *Tablets:* 5, 10 mg

Indications & dosages
➤ *Seasonal allergic rhinitis*—**Adult, child ≥ 6 yr:** 5 or 10 mg PO daily.†,‡ **Child 2-5 yr:** 2.5 mg PO daily. Max 5 mg/d.†,‡

➤ *Perennial allergic rhinitis, chronic urticaria*—**Adult, child ≥ 6 yr:** 5 or 10 mg PO daily.†,‡ **Child 6 mo-5 yr:** 2.5 mg PO daily. **Child 1-5 yr:** May increase to max of 5 mg/d in 2 divided doses.†,‡

chlordiazepoxide
Libritabs

chlordiazepoxide hydrochloride
Librium, Novo-Poxide*

Benzodiazepine; anxiolytic, anticonvulsant, sedative-hypnotic
PRC: D; CSS: IV

Available forms
chlordiazepoxide *Tablets:* 10, 25 mg; **hydrochloride** *Capsules:* 5, 10, 25 mg; *Powder for injection:* 100-mg ampule

Indications & dosages
➤ *Anxiety*—**Adult:** 5-10 mg PO tid or qid. **Child > 6 yr:** 5 mg PO bid-qid. Max 10 mg PO bid or tid.¶
➤ *Severe anxiety*—**Adult:** 20-25 mg PO tid or qid. **Elderly:** 5 mg PO bid-qid.¶
➤ *Withdrawal symptoms of acute alcoholism*—**Adult:** 50-100 mg PO, IM, or IV; repeat in 2-4 hr prn. Max 300 mg daily.¶

cholestyramine
LoCHOLEST, LoCHOLEST Light, Prevalite, Questran, Questran Light

Anion exchange resin; antilipemic, bile acid sequestrant
PRC: B

Available forms
Powder: 378-g cans, 9-g single-dose packet (1 scoop powder or single-dose packet has 4 g cholestyramine resin)

Indications & dosages
➤ *Primary hyperlipidemia or pruritus from partial bile obstruction; primary hypercholesterolemia*—**Adult:** 4 g daily or bid. Maintenance 8-16 g daily divided into 2 doses. Max 24 g daily.

cidofovir
Vistide

Nucleotide analogue; antiviral
PRC: C

Available forms
Injection: 75 mg/ml in 5-ml vial

Indications & dosages
➤ *CMV retinitis in AIDS patients*—**Adult:** 5 mg/kg IV over 1 hr in 1 dose/wk × 2 consecutive wk; then maintenance dose 5 mg/kg IV over 1 hr q 2 wk. Must give probenecid and prehydration with NSS IV at same time.†

cilostazol
Pletal

Quinolinone phosphodiesterase inhibitor; platelet aggregation inhibitor, vasodilator
PRC: C

Available forms
Tablets: 50, 100 mg

---

§ Adjust in immunocompromised patients   ¶ Adjust in debilitated patients

Indications & dosages

➤ *Intermittent claudication*—**Adult:**
100 mg PO bid ≥ 30 min ac or 2 hr pc
(am and pm). Decrease to 50 mg PO bid if
giving with drug that increases cilostazol
levels.

cimetidine
Tagamet, Tagamet HB

H₂-receptor antagonist; antiulcerative
PRC: B

Available forms

Injection: 300 mg/2 ml, 300 mg in 50 ml
NSS; *Oral liq:* 300 mg/5 ml; *Tablets:* 100,
200, 300, 400, 800 mg

Indications & dosages

➤ *Duodenal ulcer*—**Adult, child > 16 yr:**
800 mg PO hs. Or, 400 mg PO bid or
300 mg qid with meals and hs. Maintenance 400 mg hs. Parenteral treatment:
300 mg dilution in 20 ml by IV push over
> 5 min q 6 hr; or, 300 mg dilution in
50 ml IV solution over 15-20 min q 6 hr;
or, 300 mg IM q 6 hr (no dilution needed).
Max 2,400 mg daily prn. Or, 900 mg/d
(37.5 mg/hr) IV dilution in 100-1,000 ml
by continuous IV infusion.
➤ *Gastric ulceration*—**Adult:** 800 mg PO
hs, or 300 mg PO qid × ≤ 8 wk.
➤ *GERD*—**Adult:** 800 mg PO bid or
400 mg qid ac and hs × 12 wk.

ciprofloxacin
Cipro, Cipro I.V., Cipro XR

Fluoroquinolone; antibiotic
PRC: C

Available forms

Infusion (premixed): 200 mg in 100 ml
D₅W, 400 mg in 200 ml D₅W; *Injection:*
200, 400 mg; *Oral suspension:* 250,
500 mg/5 ml (after reconstitution); *Tablets (extended-release, film-coated):*
500 mg; *Tablets (film-coated):* 100, 250,
500, 750 mg

Indications & dosages

➤ *UTI*—**Adult:** 250 mg PO or 200 mg IV
q 12 hr.† Or, 500 mg (extended-release)
PO daily × 3 d.
➤ *Severe UTI; mild-to-moderate bone,
joint, skin, skin-structure infection*—
Adult: 500 mg PO × 7-14 d (≥ 4-6 wk for
bone or joint infection) or 400 mg IV q
12 hr.†
➤ *Chronic prostatitis from* Escherichia
coli *or* Proteus mirabilis—**Adult:** 500 mg
PO q 12 hr × 28 d; or, 400 mg IV over
60 min q 12 hr.†
➤ *Sinusitis*—**Adult:** 400 mg IV over
60 min q 12 hr, or 500 mg PO q 12 hr ×
10 d.†
➤ *Inhalation anthrax (postexposure)*—
Adult: Initially 400 mg q 12 hr IV until
susceptibility tests are known; then
500 mg PO bid. **Child:** 10 mg/kg q 12 hr
IV; then 15 mg/kg PO q 12 hr. Max
800 mg/d IV or 1,000 mg/d PO. **All patients:** Also 1 or 2 additional antimi-
crobials. Switch to PO treatment when

---

clinically appropriate. Treat × 60 d (IV and PO combined).

ciprofloxacin hydrochloride
Ciloxan

Fluoroquinolone; antibiotic
PRC: C

Available forms
Ophthalmic solution: 0.3% (base) in 2.5- and 5-ml containers

Indications & dosages
➤ *Corneal ulcers*—**Adult, child > 12 yr:** 2 gtt in affected eye q 15 min × 1st hr; then 2 gtt q 30 min for rest of d 1. On d 2, 2 gtt q hr. On d 3-14, 2 gtt q 4 hr.
➤ *Conjunctivitis*—**Adult, child > 12 yr:** 1 or 2 gtt in affected eye q 2 hr while awake × 1st 2 d. Then 1 or 2 gtt q 4 hr while awake × 5 d.

cisplatin (cisplatinum, CDDP)
Platinol, Platinol-AQ

Alkylating agent; antineoplastic
PRC: D

Available forms
Injection: 0.5*, 1 mg/ml

Indications & dosages
➤ *Metastatic testicular CA*—**Adult:** 20 mg/m² IV daily × 5 d. Repeat q 3 wk × 3 cycles or longer.
➤ *Metastatic ovarian CA*—**Adult:** 100 mg/m² IV; repeat q 4 wk. Or, 75-100 mg/m² IV q 4 wk with cyclophosphamide.

➤ *Bladder CA*—**Adult:** 50-70 mg/m² IV q 3-4 wk. In patients with previous antineoplastic or radiation treatment, 50 mg/m² q 4 wk.

citalopram hydrobromide
Celexa

SSRI; antidepressant
PRC: C

Available forms
Oral solution: 10 mg/5 ml; *Tablets:* 10, 20, 40 mg

Indications & dosages
➤ *Depression*—**Adult:** 20 mg PO daily, increasing to 40 mg daily after 1 wk. Max 40 mg/d. Adjust dose in elderly.‡

clarithromycin
Biaxin, Biaxin XL

Macrolide; antibiotic
PRC: C

Available forms
Suspension: 125, 250 mg/5 ml; *Tablets (extended-release):* 500 mg, 14-tablet blister pack; *Tablets (film-coated):* 250, 500 mg

Indications & dosages
➤ *Pharyngitis, tonsillitis from* Streptococcus pyogenes—**Adult:** 250 mg PO q 12 hr × 10 d.† **Child:** 15 mg/kg/d PO in divided doses q 12 hr × 10 d.†
➤ *Maxillary sinusitis from* Streptococcus pneumoniae, Haemophilus influenzae, *or* Moraxella catarrhalis—**Adult:** 500 mg PO

---

§ Adjust in immunocompromised patients   ¶ Adjust in debilitated patients

q 12 hr ×14 d or 2 extended-release tablets q 24 hr × 14 d.† **Child:** 15 mg/kg/d PO in divided doses q 12 hr × 10 d.†
➤ *MAC disease in HIV infection*—**Adult:** 500 mg PO q 12 hr.† **Child:** 7.5 mg/kg PO (max 500 mg) q 12 hr. Adult, child should take with other antimycobacterials for life.†
➤ Helicobacter pylori *infection*—**Adult:** Triple-therapy, 500 mg Biaxin with 30 mg lansoprazole and 1 g amoxicillin, all given q 12 hr × 10-14 d or 500 mg Biaxin with 20 mg omeprazole and 1 g amoxicillin, all given q 12 hr × 10 d. Or, Biaxin 500 mg with rabeprazole 20 mg and amoxicillin 1,000 mg all PO bid × 7 d. Or, dual therapy with 500 mg Biaxin q 8 hr and 40 mg omeprazole daily × 14 d.† **Child:** 15 mg/kg/d divided q 12 hr × 10 d.†
➤ *Community-acquired pneumonia due to* Chlamydia pneumoniae, Mycoplasma pneumoniae, Streptococcus pneumoniae, Haemophilus influenzae, Haemophilus parainfluenzae, *or* Moraxella catarrhalis—**Adult:** 250 mg P.O. q 12 hr × 7-14 d (for *Haemophilus influenzae,* duration of therapy is 7 d). Don't use conventional tablets to treat pneumonia caused by *Haemophilus parainfluenzae or Moraxella catarrhalis.* Or, two 500-mg extended-release tablets PO daily × 7 d for all listed organisms.† **Child:** 15 mg/kg P.O. daily divided q 12 hr × 10 d (for *C. pneumoniae, Mycoplasma pneumoniae,* or Streptococcus pneumoniae only).†
➤ *Acute exacerbations of chronic bronchitis caused by* Moraxella catarrhalis, Streptococcus pneumoniae, Haemophilus influenzae, *or* Haemophilus parainfluenzae—**Adult:** 250 mg PO q 12 hr × 7-14 d (for *Moraxella catarrhalis and Strepto-*

coccus pneumoniae only), or 500 mg PO q 12 hr × 7 d (for *Haemophilus influenzae*). Or, two 500-mg extended-release tablets PO daily × 7 d.†
➤ *Uncomplicated skin and skin-structure infections caused by* Staphylococcus aureus *or* Streptococcus pyogenes—**Adult:** 250 mg PO q 12 hr × 7-14 d.†
➤ *Acute OM caused by* Haemophilus influenzae, Moraxella catarrhalis, *or* Streptococcus pneumoniae—**Child:** 7.5 mg/kg PO q 12 hr, up to 500 mg bid.†

clindamycin hydrochloride
Cleocin, Dalacin C*

clindamycin palmitate hydrochloride
Cleocin Pediatric, Dalacin C Palmitate*

clindamycin phosphate
Cleocin Phosphate, Cleocin T, Dalacin C Phosphate*

Lincomycin derivative; antibiotic
PRC: B

Available forms
Capsules: 75, 150, 300 mg; **hydrochloride, palmitate hydrochloride** *Granules for oral solution:* 75 mg/5 ml; **phosphate** *Injection:* 150 mg base/ml, 300 mg base/2 ml, 600 mg base/4 ml, 900 mg base/6 ml; *Injection for IV infusion (in D₅W):* 300, 600, 900 mg (50 ml)

Indications & dosages
➤ *Infection*—**Adult:** 150-450 mg PO q 6 hr; or 300-600 mg IM or IV q 6, 8, or 12 hr. **Child > 1 mo:** 8-25 mg/kg PO daily

in divided doses q 6-8 hr; or 15-40 mg/kg IM or IV daily in divided doses q 6 or 8 hr.
➤ *Endocarditis prophylaxis for dental procedures in patients allergic to PCN*—**Adult:** 600 mg PO 1 hr before procedure. **Child:** 20 mg/kg PO 1 hr before procedure.
➤ *PID*—**Adult:** 900 mg IV q 8 hr with gentamicin. Continue ≥ 48 hr after symptoms improve; then switch to PO clindamycin 450 mg qid for total course of 14 d.

clomipramine hydrochloride
Anafranil

TCA; antiobsessional
PRC: C

Available forms
Capsules: 25, 50, 75 mg

Indications & dosages
➤ *OCD*—**Adult:** 25 mg PO daily with meal; increase to 100 mg daily in divided doses over 1st 2 wk. Then, increase to max 250 mg daily in divided doses with meal prn. **Child:** 25 mg PO daily with meal; increase over 1st 2 wk to max 3 mg/kg/d or 100 mg PO in divided doses, whichever is smaller. Max 3 mg/kg/d or 200 mg/d, whichever is smaller. *Note:* After adjustment, may give total doses hs.

clonazepam
Klonopin

Benzodiazepine; anticonvulsant
PRC: NR; CSS: IV

Available forms
Tablets: 0.5, 1, 2 mg

Indications & dosages
➤ *Lennox-Gastaut syndrome; atypical absence, akinetic, and myoclonic seizures*—**Adult:** 1.5 mg PO daily in 3 divided doses. Increase by 0.5-1 mg q 3 d until seizures are controlled. If given in unequal doses, give largest dose hs. Max 20 mg daily. **Child ≤ 10 yr or 30 kg:** 0.01-0.03 mg/kg PO daily (max 0.05 mg/kg daily), in 2-3 divided doses. Increase 0.25-0.5 mg q 3rd d to max maintenance dose 0.1-0.2 mg/kg/d prn.

clonidine
Catapres-TTS

clonidine hydrochloride
Catapres, Dixarit*

Centrally acting adrenergic; antihypertensive
PRC: C

Available forms
clonidine *Transdermal:* TTS-1 (releases 0.1 mg/24 hr), TTS-2 (releases 0.2 mg/24 hr), TTS-3 (releases 0.3 mg/24 hr); **hydrochloride** *Tablets:* 0.025*, 0.1, 0.2, 0.3 mg

Indications & dosages
➤ *Essential and renal HTN*—**Adult:** 0.1 mg PO bid; increase by 0.1-0.2 mg daily or q few d prn. Usual 0.2-0.8 mg daily in divided doses. Doses up to 2.4 mg daily prn. Or, transdermal patch applied to nonhairy, intact skin on upper arm or torso q 7 d, starting with 0.1-mg system; then adjust with another 0.1-mg or larger system.

clopidogrel bisulfate
Plavix

Adenosine diphosphate-induced platelet aggregation inhibitor; antiplatelet
PRC: B

Available forms
Tablets: 75 mg

Indications & dosages
➤ *Reduce atherosclerotic events in patients with recent CVA, MI, or peripheral arterial disease*—**Adult:** 75 mg PO daily.
➤ *Reduce atherosclerotic events in patients with acute coronary syndrome*—**Adult:** 300 mg PO × 1 dose; then 75 mg PO daily with aspirin 75-325 mg daily.

clorazepate dipotassium
Apo-Clorazepate*, Gen-XENE, Novo-Clopate*, Tranxene, Tranxene-SD, Tranxene T-Tab

Benzodiazepine; anxiolytic, anticonvulsant, sedative-hypnotic
PRC: D; CSS: IV

Available forms
Capsules: 3.75, 7.5, 15 mg; *Tablets:* 3.75, 7.5, 11.25, 15, 22.5 mg

Indications & dosages
➤ *Alcohol withdrawal*—**d 1:** 30 mg PO in 1 dose; then 30-60 mg PO in divided doses; d 2: 45-90 mg PO in divided doses; d 3: 22.5-45 mg PO in divided doses; d 4: 15-30 mg PO in divided doses; then reduce dose to 7.5-15 mg daily. Max 90 mg daily.

➤ *Partial seizure disorder*—**Adult, adolescent > 12 yr:** Max initial dose 7.5 mg PO tid. Increase by ≤ 7.5 mg/wk to max 90 mg daily. **Child 9-12 yr:** Max initial dose 7.5 mg PO bid. Increase by ≤ 7.5 mg/wk to max 60 mg daily.

clotrimazole
Canesten Vaginal*, Gyne-Lotrimin, Lotrimin, Mycelex, Mycelex-7, Mycelex-G, Mycelex OTC

Synthetic imidazole derivative; antifungal
PRC: B

Available forms
Combination pack: vaginal inserts 100, 200 mg and vulvar cream 1%; *Cream, topical lotion and solution, vaginal cream:* 1%; *Troche:* 10 mg; *Vaginal tablets:* 100, 200, 500 mg

Indications & dosages
➤ *Superficial fungal infect*—**Adult, child:** Apply thinly and massage into affected and surrounding area, am and pm, × 2-4 wk.
➤ *Vulvovaginal candidiasis*—**Adult:** Two 100-mg or one 200-mg vaginal tablet inserted daily hs × 3 d, or one 500-mg vaginal tablet daily hs × 1 d; or one applicator vaginal cream daily hs × 3-7 d.
➤ *Oropharyngeal candidiasis*—**Adult, child > 3 yr:** Dissolve troche over 15-30 min in mouth 5 times/d × 14 d.
➤ *Prevention of oropharyngeal candidiasis in immunocompromised patients*—**Adult, child:** Dissolve troche in mouth × 15-30 min tid during chemo or until corticosteroid therapy is reduced.

clozapine
Clozaril

Tricyclic dibenzodiazepine derivative; antipsychotic
PRC: B

Available forms
Tablets: 25, 100 mg

Indications & dosages
➤ *Schizophrenia, reduce risk of recurrent suicidal behavior in schizophrenia or schizoaffective disorders*—**Adult:** 12.5 mg PO daily or bid; adjust upward at 25-50 mg daily, to 300-450 mg daily by end of 2 wk. Don't increase subsequent dose more than 1 or 2 times/wk; max 100 mg/wk. Usually 300-600 mg daily; max 900 mg/d.

codeine phosphate
Paveral*

codeine sulfate

Opioid; analgesic, antitussive
PRC: C; CSS: II

Available forms
phosphate *Injection:* 30, 60 mg/ml; *Oral solution:* 15 mg/5 ml; *Tablets (solution):* 30, 60 mg; **sulfate** *Tablets (solution):* 15, 30, 60 mg

Indications & dosages
➤ *Pain*—**Adult:** 15-60 mg PO or 15-60 mg (phosphate) SC, IM, or IV q 4-6 hr prn. **Child > 1 yr:** 0.5 mg/kg PO, SC, or IM q 4 hr prn.

➤ *Cough*—**Adult:** 10-20 mg PO q 4-6 hr. Max 120 mg/d. **Child 6-12 yr:** 5-10 mg PO q 4-6 hr; max 60 mg/d. **Child 2-6 yr:** 2.5-5 mg PO q 4-6 hr; max 30 mg/d.

colchicine

Alkaloid; antigout drug
PRC: C (PO), D (IV)

Available forms
Injection: 1 mg (1/60 grain)/2 ml; *Tablets:* 0.5 mg (1/120 grain), 0.6 mg (1/100 grain)

Indications & dosages
➤ *Gout prevention*—**Adult:** 0.5 or 0.6 mg PO daily.
➤ *Gout prevention in surgical patient*—**Adult:** 0.5 or 0.6 mg PO tid × 3 d preop and 3 d postop.
➤ *Acute gout, acute gouty arthritis*—**Adult:** 0.5-1.2 mg PO; then 0.5-1.2 mg q 1-2 hr until relief, nausea, vomiting, or diarrhea ensue or max dose of 8 mg is reached. Don't give additional doses of drug (PO) for at least 3 d. Or, 2 mg IV; then 0.5 mg IV q 6 hr prn. Max for one IV course is 4 mg/24 h. Don't give additional doses of drug (PO or IV) for at least 7 d.

colesevelam hydrochloride
Welchol

Polymeric bile acid sequestrant; anti-lipemic
PRC: B

Available forms
Tablets: 625 mg

§ Adjust in immunocompromised patients   ¶ Adjust in debilitated patients

Indications & dosages
➤ *Adjunct to diet and exercise, either alone or with an HMG-CoA reductase inhibitor, to reduce LDL-cholesterol level in patients with primary hypercholesterolemia (Frederickson type IIa)*—**Adult:** 3 tablets (1,875 mg) PO bid with meals and liq or 6 tablets (3,750 mg) once daily with meal and liq. Daily dosage can be increased to 7 tablets (4,375 mg) for added effect.

co-trimoxazole (trimethoprim-sulfamethoxazole)
Apo-Sulfatrim*, Bactrim DS, Septra, SMZ-TMP, Sulfatrim

Sulfonamide and folate antagonist; antibiotic
PRC: C (contraindicated at term)

Available forms
Oral suspension: trimethoprim 40 mg/sulfamethoxazole 200 mg/5 ml; *Injection:* trimethoprim 16 mg/sulfamethoxazole 80 mg/ml in 5-, 10-, 20-, and 30-ml vials; *Tablets (single strength):* trimethoprim 80 mg/sulfamethoxazole 400 mg; (double strength [DS]) trimethoprim 160 mg/sulfamethoxazole 800 mg

Indications & dosages
➤ *Shigellosis or UTI from Escherichia coli, Proteus, Klebsiella, or Enterobacter*—**Adult:** 1 DS tablet PO q 12 hr × 10-14 d for UTI and × 5 d for shigellosis. For uncomplicated cystitis or acute urethral syndrome, 1 DS tablet q 12 hr × 3 d. Or, IV infusion 8-10 mg/kg/d (trimethoprim)

in 2-4 divided doses q 6, 8, or 12 hr ≤ 14 d for severe UTI. Max 960 mg trimethoprim. **Child > 2 mo:** 8 mg/kg/d (trimethoprim) PO in 2 divided doses q 12 hr (10 d for UTI; 5 d for shigellosis). Or, IV infusion 8-10 mg/kg/d (trimethoprim) in 2-4 divided doses q 6, 8, or 12 hr. Don't exceed adult dose.†
➤ *Chronic bronchitis, upper respiratory infection*—**Adult:** 160 mg trimethoprim/800 mg sulfamethoxazole PO q 12 hr × 10-14 d.†
➤ *UTI with prostatitis*—**Adult:** 160 mg trimethoprim/800 mg sulfamethoxazole PO bid × 3-6 mo.†

cyanocobalamin (vitamin B₁₂)
Anacobin*, Bedoz*, Crystamine, Crysti-12, Cyanoject

hydroxocobalamin (vitamin B₁₂)
Hydro-Cobex, Hydro-Crysti-12, LA-12

H₂O-soluble vitamin; vitamin, nutritional supplement
PRC: NR

Available forms
cyanocobalamin *Injection:* 100, 1,000 mcg/ml; *Tablets:* 100, 500, 1,000 mcg; **hydroxocobalamin** *Injection:* 1,000 mcg/ml

Indications & dosages
➤ *Vitamin B₁₂ deficiency*—**Adult:** 30 mcg hydroxocobalamin IM daily × 5-10 d. Maintenance 100-200 mcg IM q mo. **Child:** 1-5 mg hydroxocobalamin over >

---

2 wk in doses of 100 mcg IM. Maintenance 30-50 mcg/mo IM.
➤ *Pernicious anemia, vitamin B₁₂ malabsorption*—**Adult:** 1,000 mcg cyanocobalamin IM or SC daily × 6-7 d; then 1,000 mcg IM or SC daily × 5-10 d; then 100-250 mcg IM or SC q 2-4 wk. **Child:** 10-50 mcg IM or SC daily × 5-10 d; then 100-250 mcg IM or SC q 2-4 wk.
➤ *Methylmalonic aciduria*—**Neonate:** 1,000 mcg cyanocobalamin IM daily.

cyclobenzaprine hydrochloride
Flexeril

TCA derivative; skeletal muscle relaxant
PRC: B

Available forms
Tablet: 5, 10 mg

Indications & dosages
➤ *Muscle spasm*—**Adult:** Initially 5 mg PO tid, then increase to 10 mg PO tid. Max 60 mg daily; max duration 2-3 wk.‡

dalteparin sodium
Fragmin

Low-molecular-weight heparin; anticoagulant
PRC: B

Available forms
Syringe: 2,500, 5,000 anti-Factor Xa IU/0.2 ml; *Vial:* 10,000 anti-Factor Xa IU/ml

Indications & dosages
➤ *DVT prophylaxis in abdominal surgery*—**Adult:** 2,500 IU SC daily, starting 1-2 hr preop; repeat daily × 5-10 d postop.
➤ *DVT prophylaxis in hip surgery*—**Adult:** 2,500 IU SC ≤ 2 hr before surgery and 2nd dose 2,500 IU SC in pm of surgery, ≥ 6 hr after 1st dose. If surgery is in pm, omit 2nd dose on day of surgery. On 1st postop d, 5,000 IU SC daily × 5-10 d. Or, 5,000 IU SC in pm before surgery, then 5,000 IU SC daily starting in pm of day of surgery × 5-10 d postop.

darbepoetin alfa
Aranesp

Hematopoietic; antianemic
PRC: C

Available forms
Injection: 25, 40, 60, 100, 150, 200, 300, 500 mcg/ml (albumin solution) in single-dose vials

Indications & dosages
➤ *Anemia related to chronic RF*—**Adult:** 0.45 mcg/kg IV or SC once/wk. Adjust dose to avoid exceeding a target Hgb level of 12 g/dl. Dose shouldn't be increased more often than monthly. If Hgb level is increasing toward 12 g/dl, reduce dose by 25%. If it continues to increase, withhold dose until Hgb level begins to decrease, and then restart drug at a dose 25% below previous dose. If Hgb level increases by more than 1 g/dl over 2 wk, decrease dose by 25%. If increase is < 1 g/dl over 4 wk and iron stores are adequate, increase dose by 25% of previous dose. Further increases can be made at 4-wk intervals until target Hgb is reached.

---

§ Adjust in immunocompromised patients   ¶ Adjust in debilitated patients

➤ *Anemia related to chemo*—**Adult:** 2.25 mcg/kg SC once/wk. If there is less than a 1 g/dl increase in Hgb after 6 wk of therapy, increase dose up to 4.5 mcg/kg. If Hgb increases by more than 1 g/dl in a 2-wk period or if the Hgb exceeds 12 g/dl, reduce dose by approximately 25%. If Hgb exceeds 13 g/dl, withhold drug until Hgb drops to 12 g/dl, then restart at a dose approximately 25% below the previous dose.

delavirdine mesylate
Rescriptor

Nonnucleoside reverse-transcriptase inhibitor; antiretroviral
PRC: C

Available forms
Tablets: 100, 200 mg

Indications & dosages
➤ *HIV-1 infection*—**Adult:** 400 mg PO tid with other antiretrovirals.

desipramine hydrochloride
Norpramin

Dibenzazepine TCA; antidepressant
PRC: C

Available forms
Tablets (regular or film-coated): 10, 25, 50, 75, 100, 150 mg

Indications & dosages
Depression—**Adult:** 100-200 mg PO daily in divided doses or hs; increase to max 300 mg daily. **Elderly, adolescent:** 25-

100 mg PO daily in divided doses, up to max 150 mg daily prn.

desloratadine
Clarinex, Claritin Reditabs

Selective H_1-receptor antagonist; antihistamine
PRC: C

Available forms
Tablets: 5 mg; *Tablets (orally disintegrating):* 5 mg

Indications & dosages
➤ *Seasonal and perennial allergic rhinitis; chronic idiopathic urticaria*—**Adult, child ≥ 12 yr:** 5 mg PO daily.†,‡

dexamethasone (injectable)
Decadron, Hexadrol

dexamethasone acetate
Cortastat LA, Dalalone D.P., Decaject-LA, Dexasone L.A., Dexone LA, Solurex LA

dexamethasone sodium phosphate
Dalalone, Decadron Phosphate, Dexasone

Glucocorticoid; anti-inflammatory, immunosuppressant
PRC: C

Available forms
dexamethasone *Elixir:* 0.5 mg/5 ml; *Oral solution:* 0.5 mg/5 ml, 1 mg/ml; *Tablets:* 0.25, 0.5, 0.75, 1, 1.5, 2, 4, 6 mg; **acetate**

Injection: 8, 16 mg/ml suspension; **sodium phosphate** *Injection:* 4, 10, 20, 24 mg/ml

Indications & dosages
➤ *Cerebral edema*—**Adult:** 10 mg (phosphate) IV; then 4-6 mg IM q 6 hr; taper over 5-7 d.
➤ *Inflammatory conditions, allergic reactions, neoplasias*—**Adult:** 0.75-9 mg/d PO or 0.5-9 mg/d (phosphate) IM; or 4-16 mg (acetate) IM into joint or soft tissue q 1-3 wk; or 0.8-1.6 mg (acetate) into lesions q 1-3 wk.
➤ *Shock*—**Adult:** 1-6 mg/kg (phosphate) IV in 1 dose; or 40 mg IV q 2-6 hr prn.

dexamethasone (ophthalmic)
Maxidex

dexamethasone sodium phosphate
Decadron

Corticosteroid; ophthalmic anti-inflammatory
PRC: C

Available forms
dexamethasone *Ophthalmic suspension:* 0.1%; **sodium phosphate** *Ophthalmic ointment:* 0.05%; *Ophthalmic solution:* 0.1%

Indications & dosages
➤ *Uveitis, iridocyclitis, inflammatory eye conditions, corneal injury, allergic conjunctivitis, suppression of graft rejection after keratoplasty*—**Adult, child:** 1 or 2 gtt suspension or solution or 1.25-2.5 cm ointment into conjunctival sac. Initially,

drops may be used from 6 times/d to q hr or ointment applied tid or qid depending on severity. Taper as condition improves.

dexmethylphenidate hydrochloride
Focalin

Methylphenidate derivative; CNS stimulant
PRC: C; CSS: II

Available forms
Tablets: 2.5, 5, 10 mg

Indications & dosages
➤ *ADHD*—**Child 6-17 yr:** For patients who aren't taking racemic methylphenidate, 2.5 mg PO bid, at least 4 hr apart. Adjust in wkly increments of 2.5-5 mg daily, to max 20 mg daily in divided doses. For patients taking methylphenidate, starting dose is ½ current methylphenidate dosage. Max 20 mg PO daily in divided doses.

diazepam
Apo-Diazepam*, Diazepam Intensol, Valium

Benzodiazepine; anxiolytic; skeletal muscle relaxant, amnestic, anticonvulsant, sedative-hypnotic
PRC: D; CSS: IV

Available forms
Injection: 5 mg/ml; *Oral solution:* 5 mg/5 ml; 5 mg/ml; *Tablets:* 2, 5, 10 mg

Indications & dosages
➤ *Anxiety*—**Adult:** 2-10 mg PO bid-qid. Or, 2-10 mg IM or IV q 3-4 hr prn. **Elderly:**

2-2.5 mg daily or bid; increase prn. **Child
≥ 6 mo:** 1-2.5 mg PO tid or qid; increase
prn.
➤ *Muscle spasm*—**Adult:** 2-10 mg PO
bid-qid. Or, 5-10 mg IM or IV, then 5-
10 mg IM or IV q 3-4 hr prn. **Child > 30 d-
5 yr:** 1-2 mg IM or IV slowly; repeat q 3-
4 hr prn. **Child ≥ 5 yr:** 5-10 mg IM or IV q
3-4 hr prn.
➤ *Status epilepticus*—**Adult:** 5-10 mg IV
(preferred) or IM. Repeat q 10-15 min
prn, to max 30 mg. Repeat q 2-4 hr prn.
Child > 30 d-5 yr: 0.2-0.5 mg IV slowly q
2-5 min to max 5 mg. Repeat q 2-4 hr
prn. **Child ≥ 5 yr:** 1 mg IV q 2-5 min to
max 10 mg. Repeat q 2-4 hr prn.

diclofenac potassium
Cataflam

diclofenac sodium
Solaraze, Voltaren, Voltaren SR*

NSAID; antarthritic, anti-inflammatory
PRC: B

Available forms
Gel: 3%; *Suppository:* 50*, 100 mg*;
Tablets: 50 mg; *Tablets (delayed-release):*
25, 50, 75 mg; *Tablets (extended-release):*
100 mg

Indications & dosages
➤ *Ankylosing spondylitis*—**Adult:** 25 mg
PO qid (and hs prn).
➤ *OA*—**Adult:** 50 mg PO bid or tid, or
75 mg PO bid (sodium).
➤ *RA*—**Adult:** 50 mg PO tid or qid. Or,
75 mg PO bid (sodium) or 100 mg PO
daily of extended-release.

➤ *Analgesia and primary dysmenorrhea*—**Adult:** 50 mg PO tid (potassium).
➤ *Actinic keratosis*—**Adult:** Apply gel to
lesion bid.

dicyclomine hydrochloride
Antispas, Bentyl, Neoquess,
Spasmoban*

*Anticholinergic; antimuscarinic, GI anti-
spasmodic*
PRC: B

Available forms
Capsules: 10, 20 mg; *Injection:* 10 mg/ml;
Syrup: 10 mg/5 ml; *Tablets:* 20 mg

Indications & dosages
➤ *IBS, functional GI disorders*—**Adult:**
20 mg PO qid, increased to 40 mg qid, or
20 mg IM q 4-6 hr.

didanosine (ddI)
Videx, Videx EC

Purine analogue; antiviral
PRC: B

Available forms
Capsules (delayed-release): 125, 200,
250, 400 mg; *Powder for oral solution
(buffered):* 100, 167, 250 mg/packet;
Powder for oral solution (pediatric): 4-,
8-oz glass bottles contain 2, 4 g Videx, respectively; *Tablets (buffered, chewable):*
25, 50, 100, 150, 200 mg

Indications & dosages
➤ *HIV infection*—**Adult ≥ 60 kg:** 200 mg
(tablet) PO q 12 hr; or 250 mg (buffered

powder) PO q 12 hr; or 400 mg (capsule) PO daily. **Adult < 60 kg:** 125 mg (tablet) PO q 12 hr; or 167 mg (buffered powder) PO q 12 hr; or 250 mg (capsule) PO daily. **Child:** 120 mg/m² PO q 12 hr.†

digoxin
Digitek, Digoxin, Lanoxicaps, Lanoxin

Cardiac glycoside; antiarrhythmic, inotropic
PRC: C

Available forms
Capsules: 0.05, 0.1, 0.2 mg; *Elixir:* 0.05 mg/ml; *Injection:* 0.1 (pediatric), 0.25 mg/ml; *Tablets:* 0.125, 0.25 mg

Indications & dosages
➤ *HF, PSVT, atrial fibrillation and flutter—* **Adult:** Loading 0.5-1 mg IV or PO in divided doses over 24 hr; maintenance 0.125-0.5 mg IV or PO daily. **Adult > 65 yr:** Maintenance 0.125 mg PO daily. **Premature neonate:** Loading 0.015-0.025 mg/kg IV in 3 divided doses over 24 hr; maintenance 0.01 mg/kg daily, divided q 12 hr. **Neonate:** Loading 0.025-0.035 mg/kg PO, divided q 8 hr over 24 hr; IV loading 0.02-0.03 mg/kg; maintenance 0.01 mg/kg PO daily, divided q 12 hr. **Child 1 mo-2 yr:** Loading 0.035-0.06 mg/kg PO in 3 divided doses over 24 hr; IV loading 0.03-0.05 mg/kg; maintenance 0.01-0.02 mg/kg PO daily, divided q 12 hr. **Child > 2 yr:** Loading 0.02-0.04 mg/kg PO daily, divided q 8 hr over 24 hr. IV loading, 0.015-0.035 mg/kg; maintenance 0.012 mg/kg PO daily, divided q 12 hr.†

digoxin immune Fab (ovine)
Digibind, DigiFab

Antibody fragment; cardiac glycoside antidote
PRC: C

Available forms
Injection: 38-, 40-mg vial

Indications & dosages
➤ *Digitalis intoxication—***Adult, child:** Dose is highly specific. 1 vial binds about 0.5 mg of digoxin. Average dose, 10 vials.

diltiazem hydrochloride
Apo-Diltiaz*, Cardizem, Cardizem CD, Cardizem LA, Cardizem SR, CartiaXT, Dilacor XR, Diltia XT, Tiazac

Calcium channel blocker; antianginal
PRC: C

Available forms
Capsules (extended-release): 120, 180, 240, 300, 360, 420 mg; *Capsules (sustained-release):* 60, 90, 120, 180, 240, 300, 360, 420 mg; *Injection:* 5 mg/ml (25 mg and 50 mg); *Tablets:* 30, 60, 90, 120 mg

Indications & dosages
➤ *Vasospastic angina, stable angina pectoris—***Adult:** 30 mg PO tid or qid ac and hs. Adjust prn to max 360 mg/d in divided doses. Or, 120 or 180 mg (extended-release). Adjust prn to max 480 mg daily.
➤ *HTN—***Adult:** 60-120 mg PO bid (extended-release). Adjust prn to max 360 mg/d. Or, 180-240 mg daily

---

§ Adjust in immunocompromised patients   ¶ Adjust in debilitated patients

(extended-release). Adjust prn. Or, 120-240 mg (Cardizem LA) PO daily at same time each day. Adjust q 14 d to max 540 mg/d.
➤ *Atrial fibrillation or flutter, PSVT*—**Adult:** 0.25 mg/kg as IV bolus injection over 2 min. If poor response, 0.35 mg/kg IV after 15 min; then continue infusion 10 mg/hr (range 5-15 mg/hr).

diphenhydramine hydrochloride
Allerdryl*, Benadryl, Hydramine, Nytol Maximum Strength, Sominex

Ethanolamine-derivative antihistamine; antihistamine, antiemetic, antivertigo drug, antitussive, sedative-hypnotic, antidyskinetic
PRC: B

Available forms
Elixir: 12.5 mg/5 ml (14% alcohol); *Injection:* 10, 50 mg/ml; *Syrup:* 12.5 mg/5 ml; *Tablets, capsules:* 25, 50 mg; *Tablets (chewable):* 12.5 mg

Indications & dosages
➤ *Rhinitis, allergy symptoms, motion sickness, Parkinson's disease*—**Adult, child ≥ 12 yr:** 25-50 mg PO tid or qid; or 10-50 mg deep IM or IV. Max IM or IV dose 400 mg daily. **Child < 12 yr:** 5 mg/kg daily PO, deep IM, or IV in divided doses qid. Max 300 mg daily.
➤ *Sedation*—**Adult:** 25-50 mg PO or deep IM prn.
➤ *Cough*—**Adult:** 25 mg PO q 4-6 hr (max 150 mg daily). **Child 6-12 yr:** 12.5 mg PO q 4-6 hr (max 75 mg daily).

Child 2-6 yr: 6.25 mg PO q 4-6 hr (max 25 mg/d).

diphenoxylate hydrochloride and atropine sulfate
Logen, Lomanate, Lomotil, Lonox

Opiate; antidiarrheal
PRC: C; CSS: V

Available forms
Liq: 2.5 mg/5 ml (and atropine sulfate 0.025 mg/5 ml); *Tablets:* 2.5 mg (and atropine sulfate 0.025 mg)

Indications & dosages
➤ *Diarrhea*—**Adult:** 5 mg PO qid; adjust prn. **Child 2-12 yr:** 0.3-0.4 mg/kg liq form PO daily in 4 divided doses. Maintenance, initial dose reduced by up to 75% prn.

dipyridamole
IV Persantine, Persantine

Pyrimidine analogue; coronary vaso-dilator, platelet aggregation inhibitor
PRC: B

Available forms
Injection: 10 mg/2 ml; *Tablets:* 25, 50, 75 mg

Indications & dosages
➤ *Platelet adhesion inhibitor in prosthetic heart valves*—**Adult:** 75-100 mg PO qid as an adjunct to coumarin derivatives.
➤ *Alternative to exercise in CAD evaluation during thallium stress test*—**Adult:**

0.57 mg/kg IV infusion over 4 min (0.142 mg/kg/min).

dobutamine hydrochloride
Dobutrex

Adrenergic, beta₁-agonist; inotropic

PRC: B

Available forms
Injection: 12.5 mg/ml in 20-ml vials (parenteral)

Indications & dosages
➤ *To increase cardiac output resulting from organic heart disease or from cardiac surgery*—**Adult:** 2.5-15 mcg/kg/min IV infusion. Up to 40 mcg/kg/min prn (rare).

docetaxel
Taxotere

Taxoid; antineoplastic

PRC: D

Available forms
Injection: 20, 80 mg in single-dose vials

Indications & dosages
➤ *Breast CA*—**Adult:** 60-100 mg/m² IV over 1 hr q 3 wk. For patients who have febrile neutropenia, neutrophil count < 500 cells/mm³ for > 1 wk, or severe or cumulative cutaneous reactions and who started therapy at 100 mg/m², decrease to 75 mg/m². If reactions continue, decrease dose to 55 mg/m² or stop therapy. For patients initially given 60 mg/m² and without above reactions, dosage may be in-

creased. Stop therapy in patients who develop ≥ grade 3 peripheral neuropathy.‡
➤ *Non–small-cell lung CA after failure of platinum-based chemo*—**Adult:** 75 mg/m² IV over 1 h q 3 wk. For patients who experience febrile neutropenia, neutrophils < 500 cells/mm³ for > 1 wk, severe or cumulative cutaneous reactions, or other grade 3/4 nonhematologic toxicities during treatment, withhold until resolution of toxicity, then resume at 55 mg/m². Stop treatment in patients who develop ≥ grade 3 peripheral neuropathy.‡
➤ *Non–small-cell lung CA in patients who have not previously received chemo given with cisplatin*—**Adult:** 75 mg/m² IV over 1 hr immediately followed by cisplatin 75 mg/m² over 30-60 min q 3 wk. In patients whose lowest platelet count during previous therapy was < 25,000 cells/mm³, in those with febrile neutropenia, and in those with serious nonhematologic toxicity, decrease docetaxel dosage to 65 mg/m². In patients who need a further reduction, a dose of 50 mg/m² is recommended.‡

docosanol
Abreva

Bethenyl alcohol; antiviral

PRC: B

Available forms
Cream: 10%

Indications & dosages
➤ *Recurrent oral-facial herpes simplex*—**Adult, child ≥ 12 yr:** Apply topically 5 times/d starting with first symptoms;

---

§ Adjust in immunocompromised patients   ¶ Adjust in debilitated patients

continue until lesion is healed; rub in gently but completely.

docusate calcium
Surfak

docusate sodium
Colace, Diocto liquid, Diocto syrup, D-S-S

Surfactant; emollient laxative
PRC: C

Available forms
calcium *Capsules:* 240 mg; **sodium** *Capsules:* 50, 100, 250 mg; *Oral liq:* 150 mg/ 15 ml; *Syrup:* 20 mg/5 ml, 50, 60 mg/ 15 ml, 100 mg/30 ml; *Tablets:* 100 mg

Indications & dosages
➤ *Stool softener*—**Adult, child > 12 yr:** 50-500 mg PO daily until BM is normal. **Child < 3 yr:** 10-40 mg sodium PO daily. **Child 3-6 yr:** 20-60 mg sodium PO daily. **Child 6-12 yr:** 40-120 mg sodium PO daily.

dofetilide
Tikosyn

Antiarrhythmic; class III antiarrhythmic
PRC: C

Available forms
Capsules: 125, 250, 500 mcg

Indications & dosages
➤ *Maintenance of normal sinus rhythm (NSR) in patients who had symptomatic atrial fibrillation or flutter for > 1 wk; con-*
version of atrial fibrillation and flutter to NSR—**Adult:** 500 mcg PO bid if CrCl > 60 ml/min; 250 mcg PO bid if CrCl is 40-60 ml/min; 125 mcg PO bid if CrCl is 20-< 40 ml/min. Measure QTc interval before 1st dose and q 2-3 hr after each dose in hospital. If QTc interval increases > 15% or is > 500 milliseconds (550 milliseconds in ventricular conduction abnormalities) 2-3 hr after 1st dose, adjust as follows: If initial dose was 500 mcg PO bid, give 250 mcg PO bid. If initial dose was 250 mcg PO bid, give 125 mcg PO bid. If initial dose was 125 mcg PO bid, give 125 mcg PO daily. If QTc interval > 500 milliseconds (550 milliseconds in ventricular conduction abnormalities) any time after 2nd dose, stop drug.

dolasetron mesylate
Anzemet

Selective serotonin 5-HT$_3$–receptor antagonist; antinauseant, antiemetic
PRC: B

Available forms
Injection: 20 mg/ml as 12.5 mg/0.625-ml ampule or 100 mg/5-ml vial; *Tablets:* 50, 100 mg

Indications & dosages
➤ *Prevent nausea and vomiting in chemo*—**Adult:** 100 mg PO 1 hr before chemo; or 1.8 mg/kg (or fixed dose of 100 mg) IV 30 min before chemo. **Child 2-16 yr:** 1.8 mg/kg PO 1 hr before chemo; or 1.8 mg/kg IV 30 min before chemo.
➤ *Prevent postop nausea and vomiting*—**Adult:** 100 mg PO ≤ 2 hr preop; 12.5 mg

IV 15 min before anesthesia ends. **Child 2-16 yr:** 1.2 mg/kg PO ≤ 2 hr preop, max 100 mg; or, 0.35 mg/kg (max 12.5 mg) IV 15 min before anesthesia ends. *Note:* Can mix injection with apple or apple-grape juice and give PO; max 100 mg.
➤ *Postop nausea and vomiting*—**Adult:** 12.5 mg IV when symptoms occur. **Child 2-16 yr:** 0.35 mg/kg, max 12.5 mg IV when symptoms occur.

donepezil hydrochloride
Aricept

Acetylcholinesterase inhibitor; CNS drug for Alzheimer's disease
PRC: C

Available forms
Tablets: 5, 10 mg

Indications & dosages
➤ *Dementia (Alzheimer's type)*—**Adult:** 5 mg PO daily hs. After 4-6 wk, may increase to 10 mg daily.

dopamine hydrochloride
Intropin, Revimine*

Adrenergic; inotropic, vasopressor
PRC: C

Available forms
Injection: 40, 80, 160 mg/ml parenteral concentrate for injection for IV infusion; 0.8 mg/ml (200 or 400 mg), 1.6 mg/ml (400 or 800 mg), 3.2 mg/ml (800 mg) in D_5W parenteral injection for IV infusion

Indications & dosages
➤ *Shock, improve perfusion to vital organs, increase cardiac output, hypotension*—**Adult:** 1-5 mcg/kg/min IV infusion. Increase infusion by 1-4 mcg/kg/min q 10-30 min prn.

dorzolamide hydrochloride
Trusopt

Sulfonamide; antiglaucoma drug
PRC: C

Available forms
Ophthalmic solution: 2%

Indications & dosages
➤ *Increased IOP in patients with ocular HTN or open-angle glaucoma*—**Adult:** 1 gtt in affected eye tid.

doxazosin mesylate
Cardura

Alpha blocker; antihypertensive
PRC: C

Available forms
Tablets: 1, 2, 4, 8 mg

Indications & dosages
➤ *HTN*—**Adult:** 1 mg PO daily; evaluate standing and supine BP at 2-6 hr and 24 hr after dose. Increase slowly to 2 mg, 4 mg, then 8 mg daily prn. Max 16 mg.
➤ *BPH*—**Adult:** 1 mg PO daily in am or pm; may increase to 2 mg, then 4 mg, and 8 mg daily prn. Adjust q 1-2 wk.

---

§ Adjust in immunocompromised patients   ¶ Adjust in debilitated patients

doxepin hydrochloride
Adapin, Novo-Doxepin*, Sinequan, Triadapin*

TCA; antidepressant
PRC: NR

Available forms
Capsules: 10, 25, 50, 75, 100, 150 mg;
Oral concentrate: 10 mg/ml

Indications & dosages
➤ *Depression, anxiety*—**Adult:** 25-75 mg PO daily in divided doses to max 300 mg daily. Or, give entire maintenance dose daily; max 150 mg PO.

doxycycline calcium
Vibramycin

doxycycline hyclate
Apo-Doxy*, Doryx, Doxy-100, Doxy-200, Doxycin*, Doxytec*, Novo-Doxylin*, Nu-Doxycycline*, Periostat, Vibramycin, Vibramycin I.V., Vibra-Tabs

doxycycline monohydrate
Adoxa, Monodox, Vibramycin

Tetracycline; antibiotic
PRC: D

Available forms
calcium *Oral suspension:* 50 mg/5 ml;
hyclate *Capsules:* 20, 50, 100 mg; *Capsules (enteric-coated pellets):* 75, 100 mg; *Injection:* 100, 200 mg; *Tablets:* 20, 100 mg; **monohydrate** *Capsules:* 50, 100 mg; *Oral suspension:* 25 mg/5 ml; *Tablets:* 50, 75, 100 mg

Indications & dosages
➤ *Acute gonococcal infection*—200 mg PO × 1 dose followed with 100 mg at hs on day 1, then 100 mg PO bid × 3 d. Or, 300 mg PO × 1 dose; repeat 300 mg PO in 1 hr.
➤ *Infection from susceptible gram-pos and gram-neg organisms,* Rickettsia, Mycobacterium pneumoniae, Chlamydia trachomatis, *and* Borrelia burgdorferi; *psittacosis; granuloma inguinale*—**Adult, child > 8 yr or ≥ 45 kg:** 100 mg PO q 12 hr on d 1; then 100 mg PO daily; or 200 mg IV on d 1 in 1-2 infusions; then 100-200 mg IV daily. **Child > 8 yr or < 45 kg:** 4.4 mg/kg PO or IV daily in divided doses q 12 hr on d 1; then 2.2-4.4 mg/kg daily in 1-2 divided doses. Give IV infusion ≥ 1 hr.
➤ *Urethral, endocervical, or rectal infection from* C. trachomatis *or* U. urealyticum—**Adult:** 100 mg PO bid ≥ 7 d (10 d for epididymitis).
➤ *PID*—**Adult:** 100 mg IV q 12 hr; continue ≥ 2 d after symptoms improve; then 100 mg PO q 12 h × total 14 d.
➤ *Adjunct to other antibiotics for inhalation, GI, and oropharyngeal anthrax*—**Adult:** 100 mg q 12 hr IV initially until susceptibility tests are known. Switch to 100 mg PO bid when clinically appropriate. Treat × 60 d total. **Child > 8 yr and > 45 kg:** 100 mg q 12 hr IV, then switch to 100 mg PO bid when clinically appropriate. Treat × 60 d total. **Child > 8 yr and ≤ 45 kg:** 2.2 mg/kg q 12 hr IV, then switch to 2.2 mg/kg PO bid when clinically appropriate. Treat × 60 d total. **Child ≤ 8 yr:** 2.2 mg/kg 12 hr IV, then switch to 2.2 mg/kg PO bid when clinically appropriate. Treat × 60 d total.

➤ *Cutaneous anthrax*—**Adult:** 100 mg PO bid × 60 d. **Child > 8 yr and > 45 kg:** 100 mg PO q 12 hr × 60 d. **Child > 8 yr and ≤ 45 kg:** 2.2 mg/kg PO q 12 hr × 60 d. **Child ≤ 8 yr:** 2.2 mg/kg q 12 hr PO × 60 d.¶

➤ *Periodontitis*—**Adult:** 20 mg (Periostat) PO bid > 1 hr before or 2 hr after am and pm meals and after scaling and root planing. Effective for 9 mo.

droperidol
Inapsine

Dopamine blocker, butyrophenone derivative; antipsychotic, neuroleptic
PRC: C

Available forms
Injection: 2.5 mg/ml in 1-, 2-ml ampule and 2-ml vials

Indications & dosages
➤ *Premedication*—**Adult, child > 12 yr:** 2.5-10 mg IM 30-60 min preop. **Child 2-12 yr:** 1-1.5 mg/9-11 kg IM. Adjust dose in elderly and patients taking depressants.¶

➤ *Induction as adjunct to general anesthesia*—**Adult, child > 12 yr:** 2.5 mg/9-11 kg IV. Maintenance 1.25-2.5 mg, usually IV. **Child 2-12 yr:** 1-1.5 mg/9-11 kg IV.

➤ *Diagnostic procedures (without general anesthetic)*—**Adult, child > 12 yr:** 2.5-10 mg IM 30-60 min before procedure. May give more doses of 1.25-2.5 mg, usually IV.

➤ *Adjunct to regional anesthesia when more sedation needed*—**Adult:** 2.5-5 mg IM or IV.

drotrecogin alfa (activated)
Xigris

Recombinant human activated protein C; anti-infective
PRC: C

Available forms
Injection: 5-, 20-mg vials

Indications & dosages
➤ *Severe sepsis*—**Adult:** 24 mcg/kg/hr IV infusion × 96 hr.

dutasteride
Avodart

5-Alpha-reductase enzyme inhibitor; BPH drug
PRC: X

Available forms
Capsules: 0.5 mg

Indications & dosages
➤ *Symptomatic BPH*—**Adult:** 0.5 mg PO daily.

efavirenz
Sustiva

Nonnucleoside, reverse transcriptase inhibitor; antiretroviral
PRC: C

Available forms
Capsules: 50, 100, 200 mg; *Tablets:* 600 mg

---

§ Adjust in immunocompromised patients   ¶ Adjust in debilitated patients

Indications & dosages
➤ *HIV-1 infection, given with protease inhibitor or nucleoside analogue reverse transcriptase inhibitor*—**Adult:** 600 mg PO daily. **Child ≥ 3 yr or ≥ 40 kg:** 600 mg PO daily. **Child ≥ 3 yr or 10 kg to < 40 kg:** If 10 to < 15 kg, give 200 mg PO daily; 15 to < 20 kg, 250 mg PO daily; 20 to < 25 kg, 300 mg PO daily; 25 to < 32.5 kg, 350 mg PO daily; 32.5 to < 40 kg, 400 mg PO daily.

eflornithine hydrochloride
Vaniqa

Ornithine decarboxylase inhibitor; hair growth retardant
PRC: C

Available forms
Cream: 13.9%

Indications & dosages
➤ *Reduction of unwanted facial hair (women)*—**Adult, child ≥ 12 yr:** Apply thin layer to affected facial areas and adjacent areas under chin and rub in thoroughly bid, at least 8 hr apart.

eletriptan hydrobromide
Relpax

Serotonin 5-HT₁ receptor agonist; anti-migraine
PRC: C

Available forms
Tablets: 20, 40 mg

Indications & dosages
➤ *Migraines*—**Adult:** 20-40 mg PO taken at first sign of migraine attack. If headache recurs after initial relief, may repeat dose in ≥ 2 hr. Max 80 mg/daily.

enalaprilat

enalapril maleate

ACE inhibitor; antihypertensive
PRC: C (D, 2nd and 3rd trimesters)

Available forms
enalaprilat *Injection:* 1.25 mg/ml; **enalapril maleate** *Tablets:* 2.5, 5, 10, 20 mg

Indications & dosages
➤ *HTN*—**Adult:** Patients not on diuretics: 2.5-5 mg PO daily, then adjust prn. Range 10-40 mg daily in 1 dose or 2 divided doses. Or, 1.25 mg IV q 6 hr over 5 min. Patients on diuretics: 2.5 mg PO daily. Or, 0.625 mg IV over 5 min; repeat in 1 hr prn, then 1.25 mg IV q 6 hr.†
➤ *IV to PO treatment*—**Adult:** 5 mg PO daily; for patients who had been receiving 0.625 mg IV q 6 hr, then 2.5 mg PO daily.†
➤ *PO to IV treatment*—**Adult:** 1.25 mg IV over 5 min q 6 hr.†

enoxaparin sodium
Lovenox

Low-molecular-weight heparin; anticoagulant
PRC: B

Available forms
Injection: 30 mg/0.3 ml, 40 mg/0.4 ml, 60 mg/0.6 ml, 80 mg/0.8 ml, 100 mg/1 ml, 120 mg/0.8 ml, 150 mg/1 ml

Indications & dosages
➤ *Prevent DVT, which may lead to PE, following hip or knee replacement surgery*—**Adult:** 30 mg SC q 12 hr × 7-10 d. Initial dose between 12 and 24 hr postop if hemostasis is established.
➤ *Prevent DVT, which may lead to PE, after abdominal surgery*—**Adult:** 40 mg SC daily × 7-10 d. Initial dose 2 hr before surgery.
➤ *Prevent ischemic complications of unstable angina and non-Q-wave MI, when given with aspirin*—**Adult:** 1 mg/kg SC q 12 hr × 2-8 d, with aspirin PO.
➤ *Medical patients at risk of embolism from decreased mobility during acute illness.*—**Adult:** 40 mg daily SC × 6-11 d. Up to 14 d has been well tolerated.
➤ *DVT inpatient treatment with or without PE; administration with warfarin sodium*—**Adult:** 1 mg/kg SC q 12 hr; or 1.5 mg/kg SC daily × 5-7 d until INR is 2-3. Warfarin sodium starts ≤ 72 hr after enoxaparin injection.
➤ *DVT outpatient treatment without PE, administration with warfarin sodium*—**Adult:** 1 mg/kg SC q 12 hr × 5-7 d until INR is 2-3. Warfarin sodium starts ≤ 72 hr after enoxaparin injection.

entacapone
Comtan

Catechol-O-methyltransferase inhibitor; antiparkinsonian
PRC: C

Available forms
Tablets: 200 mg

Indications & dosages
➤ *Parkinson's disease*—**Adult:** 200 mg PO with each dose of levodopa-carbidopa. Max 8 doses/d (1,600 mg/d).

epinephrine (adrenaline)
Adrenalin, Bronkaid Mist, Bronkaid Mistometer*, Primatene Mist

epinephrine bitartrate
AsthmaHaler Mist, Bronkaid Suspension Mist

epinephrine hydrochloride
Adrenalin Chloride, AsthmaNefrin*, EpiPen, EpiPen Jr., Racepinephrine, Sus-Phrine, Vaponefrin

Adrenergic; bronchodilator, vasopressor, cardiac stimulant
PRC: C

Available forms
Aerosol inhalation: 160, 200, 220, 250 mcg/metered spray; *Injection:* 0.01 (1:100,000), 0.1 (1:10,000), 0.5 (1:2,000), 1 (1:1,000) mg/ml parenteral, 5 mg/ml (1:200) parenteral suspension; *Nebulizer inhalation:* 1% (1:100)*, 1.25%*, 2.25%*

---

§ Adjust in immunocompromised patients   ¶ Adjust in debilitated patients

Indications & dosages
➤ *Bronchospasm, hypersensitivity reactions, anaphylaxis*—**Adult:** 0.1-0.5 ml 1:1,000 SC or IM. Repeat q 10-15 min prn. Or, 0.1-0.25 ml 1:1,000 IV over 5-10 min. **Child:** 0.01 ml (10 mcg) 1:1,000/kg SC; repeat q 20 min-4 hr prn. Or, 0.004-0.005 ml/kg 1:200 (Sus-Phrine) SC; repeat q 8-12 hr prn.
➤ *Asthma attacks*—**Adult, child ≥ 4 yr:** 160-250 mcg (metered aerosol), equivalent to 1 inhalation, repeated × 1 dose prn, after 1 min; no subsequent doses for ≥ 3 hr. Or, 1% (1:100) solution epinephrine or 2.25% solution racepinephrine by hand-bulb nebulizer as 1-3 deep inhalations; repeat q 3 hr prn.
➤ *Cardiac arrest*—**Adult:** 0.5-1 mg IV. Repeat q 3-5 min prn. Higher-dose epinephrine: 3-5 mg (about 0.1 mg/kg) repeated q 3-5 min. **Child:** 0.01 mg/kg (0.1 ml/kg 1:10,000 injection) IV. ET tube: 0.1 mg/kg (0.1 ml/kg 1:1,000 injection) diluted in 1-2 ml ½ NSS or NSS. Subsequent IV or intratracheal doses 0.1-0.2 mg/kg (0.1-0.2 ml/kg 1:1,000 injection). May repeat q 3-5 min.

eplerenone
Inspra

Aldosterone receptor antagonist; antihypertensive
PRC: B

Available forms
Tablets: 25, 50, 100 mg

Indications & dosages
➤ *HTN*—**Adult:** 50 mg PO daily. Increase to 50 mg PO bid after 4 wk, if response is inadequate. Max 100 mg daily.

epoetin alfa (erythropoietin)
Epogen, Procrit

Glycoprotein; antianemic
PRC: C

Available forms
Injection: 2,000, 3,000, 4,000, 10,000 units/ml; multidose vials of 10,000, 20,000 units/ml

Indications & dosages
➤ *Anemia in end-stage renal disease*—**Adult:** 50-100 units/kg IV 3 times/wk (SC or IV in nonhemodialysis patients). Reduce dose when target Hct is reached or Hct rises > 4 points in 2-wk period. Increase dose if Hct doesn't increase by 5-6 points after 8 wk of treatment.
➤ *HIV-infected patients with anemia secondary to zidovudine treatment*—**Adult:** 100 units/kg IV or SC 3 times/wk × 8 wk or target Hgb level is reached. After 8 wk, may increase by 50-100 units/kg IV or SC 3 times/wk prn. After 4-8 wk, may increase in increments of 50-100 units/kg 3 times/wk; max 300 units/kg IV or SC 3 times/wk.
➤ *Anemia secondary to chemo*—**Adult:** 150 units/kg SC 3 times/wk × 8 wk or target Hgb level is reached.

---

eprosartan mesylate
Teveten

Angiotensin II-receptor antagonist; anti-hypertensive
PRC: C (D, 2nd and 3rd trimesters)

Available forms
Tablets: 400, 600 mg

Indications & dosages
➤ *HTN*—**Adult:** 600 mg PO daily. Range 400-800 mg daily in 1 dose or divided bid.

ertapenem
Invanz

Carbapenem; anti-infective
PRC: B

Available forms
Injection: 1 g

Indications & dosages
➤ *Complicated intra-abdominal infections caused by* Escherichia coli, Clostridium clostridiiforme, Eubacterium lentum, Peptostreptococcus species, Bacteroides fragilis, B. distasonis, B. ovatus, B. thetaiotaomicron, B. uniformis—**Adult:** 1 g IV or IM daily × 5-14 d.†
➤ *Complicated skin and skin-structure infections caused by* Staphylococcus aureus (methicillin-susceptible strains), Streptococcus pyogenes, Escherichia coli, Peptostreptococcus species—**Adult:** 1 g IV or IM daily × 7-14 d.†
➤ *Community-acquired pneumonia caused by* Streptococcus pneumoniae (penicillin-susceptible strains), Haemophilus influenzae *(beta-lactamase–negative strains),* Moraxella catarrhalis—**Adults:** 1 g IV or IM daily × 10-14 d. If clinical improvement occurs after at least 3 d of treatment, appropriate oral therapy may be used to complete full course of therapy.†
➤ *Complicated UTIs, including pyelonephritis caused by* Escherichia coli, Klebsiella pneumoniae—**Adult:** 1 g IV or IM daily × 10-14 d. After at least 3 d of treatment, if clinical improvement occurs, appropriate oral therapy may be used to complete full course of therapy.†
➤ *Acute pelvic infections including postpartum endomyometritis, septic abortion, and postsurgical gynecologic infections caused by* Streptococcus agalactiae, Escherichia coli, B. fragilis, Porphyromonas asaccharolyticus, Peptostreptococcus species, Prevotella bivia—**Adult:** 1 g IV or IM daily × 3-10 d.†

erythromycin base
E-Mycin, Eramycin, Eryc, Robimycin

erythromycin estolate
Ilosone

erythromycin ethylsuccinate
EryPed, EryPed 200

erythromycin lactobionate
Erythrocin

erythromycin stearate
Erythrocin Stearate

Erythromycin; antibiotic
PRC: B

Available forms
base *Capsules (delayed-release, enteric-coated):* 250 mg; *Tablets (enteric-coated):* 250, 333, 500 mg; *Tablets (filmtabs):* 250, 500 mg; **estolate** *Capsules:* 250 mg; *Oral suspension:* 125, 250 mg/5 ml; *Tablets:* 500 mg; **ethylsuccinate** *Oral suspension:* 200, 400 mg/5 ml; 100 mg/2.5 ml; *Tablets (chewable):* 200 mg; *Tablets (filmcoated):* 400 mg; **lactobionate** *Injection:* 500-mg, 1-g vial; **stearate** *Tablets (filmcoated):* 250, 500 mg

Indications & dosages
➤ *PID from* Neisseria gonorrhoeae— **Adult:** 500 mg IV (lactobionate) q 6 hr × 3 d, then 250 mg (base, estolate, stearate); or 400 mg (ethylsuccinate) PO q 6 hr × 7 d.
➤ *Respiratory tract, skin, soft-tissue infection—***Adult:** 250-500 mg (base, estolate, stearate) PO q 6 hr; or 400-800 mg (ethylsuccinate) PO q 6 hr; or 15-20 mg/kg IV daily (lactobionate) continuous infusion or divided doses q 6 hr × 10 d. **Child:** 30-50 mg/kg (PO salts) PO daily, divided doses q 6 hr; or 15-20 mg/kg IV daily, divided doses q 4-6 hr × 10 d.

escitalopram oxalate
Lexapro

SSRI; antidepressant
PRC: C

Available forms
Solution: 5 mg/5 ml; *Tablets:* 5, 10, 20 mg

Indications & dosages
➤ *Major depressive disorder—***Adult:** 10 mg PO daily; increase to 20 mg prn, after ≥ 1 wk. **Elderly:** 10 mg PO daily.‡

esmolol hydrochloride
Brevibloc

Beta blocker; antiarrhythmic
PRC: C

Available forms
Injection: 10-mg/ml vial; 250-mg/ml ampule

Indications & dosages
➤ *SVT, atrial fibrillation or flutter, noncompensatory ST—***Adult:** Loading dose 500 mcg/kg/min IV infusion over 1 min; then 4-min maintenance infusion of 50 mcg/kg/min. If no response in 5 min, repeat loading dose, then maintenance infusion of 100 mcg/kg/min × 4 min. Repeat loading dose and increase maintenance infusion by 50-mcg/kg/min increments. Max maintenance infusion for tachycardia 25-200 mcg/kg/min.
➤ *Periop, postop tachycardia or HTN—***Adult:** Periop treatment of tachycardia or HTN: 80 mg (about 1 mg/kg) IV bolus over 30 sec; then 150 mcg/kg/min IV infusion prn. Adjust rate prn. Max 300 mcg/kg/min.

esomeprazole magnesium
Nexium

Proton pump inhibitor, s-isomer of omeprazole; gastroesophageal agent
PRC: B

Available forms
Capsules (delayed-release containing enteric-coated pellets): 20, 40 mg (supplied as 22.3 or 44.5 mg esomeprazole magnesium)

Indications & dosages
➤ *GERD, healing of erosive esophagitis*—**Adult:** 20 or 40 mg PO daily × 4-8 wk.‡
➤ *Maintenance of healing in erosive esophagitis*—**Adult:** 20 mg PO daily × ≤ 6 mo.‡
➤ *Symptomatic GERD*—**Adult:** 20 mg PO daily × 4 wk. If symptoms continue, treatment may continue × 4 more wk.‡
➤ *Eradication of* Helicobacter pylori *(with other medication) to reduce duodenal ulcer recurrence*—**Adult:** 40 mg PO daily with amoxicillin 1,000 mg PO bid and clarithromycin 500 mg PO bid, all × 10 d.‡

esterified estrogens
Estratab, Menest, Neo-Estrone*

Estrogen; estrogen replacement, antineoplastic
PRC: X

Available forms
Tablets, tablets (film-coated): 0.3, 0.625, 1.25, 2.5 mg

Indications & dosages
➤ *Inoperable prostate CA*—**Men:** 1.25-2.5 mg PO tid.
➤ *Breast CA*—**Men and postmenopausal women:** 10 mg PO tid ≥ 3 mo.

➤ *Female hypogonadism*—**Women:** 2.5-7.5 mg daily in divided doses in cycles of 20 d on, 10 d off.
➤ *Female castration, primary ovarian failure*—**Women:** 1.25 mg daily in cycles of 3 wk on, 1 wk off. Adjust prn.
➤ *Osteoporosis prevention*—**Postmenopausal women:** 0.3-1.25 mg daily.

estradiol
Alora, Climara, Esclim, Estraderm, Vivelle, Vivelle Dot

estradiol cypionate
depGynogen, Depo-Estradiol, DepoGen

estradiol valerate
Climara, Delestrogen, Dioval, Estradiol L.A., Estra-L 40, Gynogen L.A., Menaval-20

Estrogen; estrogen replacement, antineoplastic
PRC: X

Available forms
estradiol *Tablets (micronized):* 0.5, 1, 2 mg; *Transdermal:* 0.025 mg, 0.0375 mg, 0.05, 0.075, 0.1 mg/24 hr, 4 mg/10 cm² (delivers 0.05 mg/24 hr), 8 mg/20 cm² (delivers 0.1 mg/24 hr); *Vaginal cream (in non-liquefying base):* 0.1 mg/g; **cypionate** *Injection (in oil):* 5 mg/ml; **valerate** *Injection (in oil):* 10, 20, 40 mg/ml

Indications & dosages
➤ *Menopausal symptoms, female hypogonadism, female castration, primary ovarian failure*—**Women:** 1-2 mg PO (estradiol) daily in cycles of 21 d on, 7 d

off, or cycles of 5 d on, 2 d off. Or, 0.025-mg/d (Esclim) or 0.05-mg/d system (Estraderm) applied twice/wk. Or, 0.05-mg/d system (Climara) once/wk. Or, 1-5 mg (cypionate) IM q 3-4 wk, or 10-20 mg (valerate) IM q 4 wk prn.
➤ *Breast CA*—**Men and postmenopausal women:** 10 mg PO (estradiol) tid × 3 mo.
➤ *Prostate CA*—**Men:** 30 mg IM (valerate) q 1-2 wk; or 1-2 mg PO (estradiol) tid.
➤ *Osteoporosis prevention*—**Postmenopausal women:** 0.025-mg/d system (Alora, Vivelle, Vivelle Dot). Or, 0.05-mg/d system (Estraderm) applied to clean, dry area of trunk twice/wk. Or, 0.025-mg/d system (Climara) once/wk.

estrogens, conjugated (estrogenic substances, conjugated)
C.E.S.*, Premarin, Premarin Intravenous Cenestin

Estrogen; estrogen replacement, antineoplastic, antiosteoporotic
PRC: X

Available forms
Injection: 25 mg/5 ml; *Tablets:* 0.3, 0.45, 0.625, 0.9, 1.25, 2.5 mg; *Vaginal cream:* 0.625 mg/g

Indications & dosages
➤ *Abnormal uterine bleeding*—**Women:** 25 mg IV or IM; repeat in 6-12 hr prn.
➤ *Female castration, primary ovarian failure*—**Women:** 1.25 mg PO daily in cycles of 3 wk on, 1 wk off.

➤ *Osteoporosis*—**Postmenopausal women:** 0.625 mg PO daily in cycles of 3 wk on, 1 wk off.

estropipate (piperazine estrone sulfate)
Ogen, Ortho-Est

Estrogen; estrogen replacement
PRC: X

Available forms
Tablets: 0.75, 1.5, 3, 6 mg; *Vaginal cream:* 1.5 mg/g

Indications & dosages
➤ *Primary ovarian failure, female castration, female hypogonadism*—**Women:** 1.25-7.5 mg PO daily × 1st 3 wk, then rest × 8-10 d. If no bleeding occurs by end of rest, repeat cycle.
➤ *Vasomotor menopausal symptoms*—**Women:** 0.625-5 mg PO daily in cycles of 3 wk on, 1 wk off.
➤ *Prevention of osteoporosis*—**Women:** 0.625 mg PO daily × 25 d of 31-d cycle.

etanercept
Enbrel

Fusion protein; antirheumatic
PRC: B

Available forms
Injection: 25-mg single-use vial

Indications & dosages
➤ *RA, psoriatic arthritis*—**Adult:** 25 mg SC 2 times/wk, 72-96 hr apart.

➤ *Juvenile RA*—**Child 4-17 yr:** 0.4 mg/kg (max 25 mg/dose) SC 2 times/wk, 72-96 hr apart.

ethambutol hydrochloride
Etibi*, Myambutol

Semisynthetic antituberculotic; antituberculotic
PRC: B

Available forms
Tablets: 100, 400 mg

Indications & dosages
➤ *Pulmonary TB*—**Adult, child > 13 yr:** Initial treatment (no previous antitubercular treatment), 15 mg/kg PO daily. Retreatment: 25 mg/kg PO daily × 60 d (or smears, cultures negative) with at least 1 other antituberculotic; then decrease to 15 mg/kg/d.

etodolac
Lodine

NSAID; antarthritic
PRC: C

Available forms
Capsules: 200, 300 mg; *Tablets:* 400, 500 mg; *Tablets (extended-release):* 400, 500, 600 mg

Indications & dosages
➤ *Pain*—**Adult:** 200-400 mg PO q 6-8 hr prn; max 1,200 mg daily. Patients ≤ 60 kg, max 20 mg/kg/d.

ezetimibe
Zetia

Selective cholesterol absorption inhibitor; antihypercholesterolemic
PRC: C

Available forms
Tablets: 10 mg

Indications & dosages
➤ *Adjunct to diet and exercise to reduce cholesterol, LDL, and apolipoprotein-B levels in patients with primary hypercholesterolemia, alone or combined with HMG-CoA reductase inhibitors or bile acid sequestrants; adjunct to other lipid-lowering drugs in patients with homozygous familial hypercholesterolemia; adjunct to diet in patients with homozygous sitosterolemia to reduce sitosterol and campesterol levels*—**Adult:** 10 mg PO daily.

famciclovir
Famvir

Synthetic acyclic guanine derivative; antiviral
PRC: B

Available forms
Tablets: 125, 250, 500 mg

Indications & dosages
➤ *Herpes zoster (shingles)*—**Adult:** 500 mg PO q 8 hr × 7 d.†
➤ *Recurrent genital herpes*—**Adult:** 125 mg PO bid × 5 d. Start when symptoms occur.†

---

§ Adjust in immunocompromised patients   ¶Adjust in debilitated patients

famotidine
Pepcid, Pepcid AC, Pepcid RPD

H₂-receptor antagonist; antiulcerative
PRC: B

Available forms
Gelcaps: 10 mg; *Injection:* 10 mg/ml; *Powder for oral suspension:* 40 mg/ml after reconstitution; *Premixed injection:* 20 mg/50 ml NSS; *Tablets:* 10, 20, 40 mg; *Tablets (chewable):* 10 mg; *Tablets (orally disintegrating):* 20, 40 mg

Indications & dosages
➤ *Duodenal ulcer*—**Adult:** 40 mg PO q hs, or 20 mg PO bid. Maintenance 20 mg PO q hs.
➤ *Benign gastric ulcer*—**Adult:** 40 mg PO q hs × 8 wk.
➤ *GERD*—**Adult:** 20 mg PO bid ≤ 6 wk.
➤ *Esophagitis from GERD*—**Adult:** 20-40 mg bid × ≤ 12 wk.
➤ *Heartburn*—**Adult:** 10 mg (Pepcid AC) PO 1 hr ac (prevention) or 10 mg (Pepcid AC) PO with H₂O for symptoms. Max 20 mg daily. Don't take daily > 2 wk.
➤ *Hospitalized patient who has ulcerations or hypersecretory conditions, or who can't take drugs PO*—**Adult:** 20 mg IV q 12 hr.

felodipine
Plendil, Renedil*

Calcium channel blocker; antihypertensive
PRC: C

Available forms
Tablets (extended-release): 2.5, 5, 10 mg

Indications & dosages
➤ *HTN*—**Adult:** 5 mg PO daily. Adjust q 2 wk prn. Max 20 mg daily. **Elderly > 65 yr:** 2.5 mg PO daily. Max 10 mg daily.‡

fenofibrate (micronized)
Lofibra, Tricor

Fibric acid derivative; antihyperlipidemic
PRC: C

Available forms
Capsules: 67, 134, 200 mg; *Tablets:* 54, 160 mg

Indications & dosages
➤ *Hypertriglyceridemia*—**Adult:** 54-160 mg PO daily. Based on response, increase dose at 4- to 8-wk intervals to max dose 160 mg daily.†
➤ *Primary hypercholesterolemia or mixed hyperlipidemia*—**Adult:** 160 mg PO daily.† **Elderly:** Start treatment at 54 mg daily and increase only after effects on renal function and triglyceride levels have been evaluated at this dose.

fentanyl citrate
Sublimaze

fentanyl transdermal system
Duragesic

fentanyl transmucosal
Actiq

---

*Canadian   † Adjust in renal impairment   ‡ Adjust in liver impairment

Opioid agonist; analgesic, adjunct to anesthesia, anesthetic
PRC: C; CSS: II

Available forms

Injection: 50 mcg/ml; *Lozenges:* 200, 400, 600, 800, 1,200, 1,600 mcg; *Transdermal system:* 25, 50, 75, 100 mcg/hr

Indications & dosages

➤ *Preop*—**Adult:** 50-100 mcg IM 30-60 min preop.
➤ *Adjunct to general anesthesia*—**Adult:** Low-dose, 2 mcg/kg IV; moderate, 2-20 mcg/kg IV, then 25-100 mcg IV prn; high, 20-50 mcg/kg IV, then 25 mcg to ½ initial loading dose IV prn.
➤ *Adjunct to regional anesthesia*—**Adult:** 50-100 mcg IM or IV over 1-2 min prn.
➤ *Induction and maintenance of anesthesia*—**Child 2-12 yr:** 2-3 mcg/kg IV.
➤ *Postop*—**Adult:** 50-100 mcg IM q 1-2 hr prn.
➤ *Chronic pain*—**Adult:** 1 transdermal system applied to upper torso skin not irritated or irradiated. Initially, 25-mcg/hr system × 72 hr (q 48 hr prn); adjust dose prn.
➤ *Breakthrough cancer pain in opioid-tolerant patients (Actiq only):* Initially 200-mcg lozenge; if no relief, repeat dose 15 min after completion of first lozenge. Max 2 lozenges per breakthrough pain episode. May increase prn until single lozenge provides adequate analgesia per breakthrough pain episode, but limit use of lozenge to ≤ 4 daily.

ferrous gluconate
Fergon, Simron

Oral iron supplement; hematinic
PRC: A

Available forms

100 mg ferrous gluconate = 11.6 mg elemental iron
Tablets: 240, 325 mg

Indications & dosages

➤ *Iron deficiency*—**Adult:** 100-200 mg (2-3 mg/kg) elemental iron PO in 3 divided doses. **Child 2-12 yr:** 50-100 mg (1-1.5 mg/kg) elemental iron PO in 3-4 divided doses. **Child 6 mo-2 yr:** Up to 6 mg/kg/d PO in 3-4 divided doses. **Infant:** 10-25 mg in 3-4 divided doses PO.

ferrous sulfate
Apo-Ferrous Sulfate*, Feosol, Mol-Iron

ferrous sulfate, dried
Feosol

Oral iron supplement; hematinic
PRC: A

Available forms

Ferrous sulfate = 20% elemental iron; dried and powdered, about 32% elemental iron
Capsules: 250 mg; *Capsules (extended-release):* 160 mg (dried); *Drops:* 75 mg/0.6 ml, 125 mg/ml; *Elixir:* 220/5 ml; *Syrup:* 90 mg/5 ml; *Tablets:* 187, 324, 325, 200 (dried) mg; *Tablets (extended-release):* 160 mg (dried), 525 mg

---

§ Adjust in immunocompromised patients   ¶ Adjust in debilitated patients

Indications & dosages

➤ *Iron deficiency*—**Adult:** 100-200 mg (2-3 mg/kg) elemental iron PO in 3 divided doses. **Child 2-12 yr:** 50-100 mg (1-1.5 mg/kg) elemental iron PO in 3-4 divided doses. **Child 6 mo-2 yr:** Up to 6 mg/kg/d PO in 3-4 divided doses. **Infant:** 10-25 mg in 3-4 divided doses PO.

fexofenadine
Allegra

H₁-receptor antagonist; antihistamine

H_1-receptor antagonist; antihistamine
PRC: C

Available forms

Tablets: 30, 60, 180 mg

Indications & dosages

➤ *Seasonal allergic rhinitis*—**Adult, child ≥ 12 yr:** 60 mg PO bid or 180 mg PO once daily.† **Child 6-11 yr:** 30 mg PO bid.†
➤ *Chronic idiopathic urticaria*—**Adult, child ≥ 12 yr:** 60 mg PO bid.† **Child 6-11 yr:** 30 mg PO bid.†

filgrastim (granulocyte colony-stimulating factor; G-CSF)
Neupogen

Biologic response modifier; colony-stimulating factor
PRC: C

Available forms

Injection: 300 mcg/ml

Indications & dosages

➤ *Decrease infection in patients with non-myeloid malignant disease on myelosuppressive antineoplastics*—**Adult, child:** 5 mcg/kg/d IV or SC ≥ 24 hr after cytotoxic chemo. Increase by 5 mcg/kg for each chemo cycle based on neutrophil count.
➤ *Decrease infection in patients with non-myeloid malignant disease on myelosuppressive antineoplastics followed by bone marrow transplantation*—**Adult, child:** 10 mcg/kg/d IV or SC ≥ 24 hr after cytotoxic chemo and bone marrow infusion. Adjust dose based on neutrophil response.
➤ *Congenital neutropenia*—**Adult:** 6 mcg/kg SC bid. Adjust dose prn.

finasteride
Propecia, Proscar

Steroid (synthetic 4-azasteroid) derivative; androgen synthesis inhibitor
PRC: X

Available forms

Tablets: 1, 5 mg

Indications & dosages

➤ *Symptomatic BPH*—**Adult:** 5 mg (Proscar) PO daily.
➤ *Male pattern hair loss (man)*—**Adult:** 1 mg (Propecia) PO daily.

flecainide acetate
Tambocor

Benzamide derivative local anesthetic; ventricular antiarrhythmic
PRC: C

Available forms

Tablets: 50, 100, 150 mg

Indications & dosages

➤ *PSVT; paroxysmal atrial fibrillation, flutter; supraventricular arrhythmias—* **Adult:** 50 mg PO q 12 hr. Increase 50 mg bid q 4 d prn. Max 300 mg/d.
➤ *Life-threatening ventricular arrhythmias—***Adult:** 100 mg PO q 12 hr. Increase 50 mg bid q 4 d prn. Max 400 mg daily.†

fluconazole
Diflucan

Bis-triazole derivative; antifungal
PRC: C

Available forms

Injection: 200 mg/100 ml; 400 mg/200 ml; *Powder for oral suspension:* 10, 40 mg/ ml; *Tablet:* 50, 100, 150, 200 mg

Indications & dosages

➤ *Oropharyngeal, esophageal candidiasis—***Adult:** 200 mg PO or IV d 1; then 100 mg daily. Continue ≥ 2 wk after symptoms end. **Child:** 6 mg/kg on d 1; then 3 mg/kg ≥ 2 wk.†
➤ *Vaginal candidiasis—***Adult:** 150 mg PO × 1 dose.†
➤ *Systemic candidiasis—***Adult:** Up to 400 mg PO or IV daily. Continue ≥ 2 wk after symptoms end.†
➤ *Cryptococcal meningitis—***Adult:** 400 mg PO or IV on d 1; then 200 mg daily. Continue 10-12 wk after CSF cultures are negative.†

fludrocortisone acetate
Florinef

Mineralocorticoid, glucocorticoid; mineralocorticoid replacement therapy
PRC: C

Available forms

Tablets: 0.1 mg

Indications & dosages

➤ *Adrenal insufficiency, salt-losing adrenogenital syndrome—***Adult:** 0.1-0.2 mg PO daily. Decrease to 0.05 mg daily if transient HTN occurs. **Child:** 0.05-0.1 mg PO daily.
➤ *Orthostatic hypotension in diabetic patients, orthostatic hypotension—***Adult:** 0.1-0.4 mg PO daily.

flumazenil
Romazicon

Benzodiazepine antagonist; antidote
PRC: C

Available forms

Injection: 0.1 mg/ml in 5-, 10-ml multi-dose vials

Indications & dosages

➤ *Reversal of sedative effects of benzodiazepines—***Adult:** 0.2 mg IV over 15 sec. After 45 sec, repeat at 1-min intervals until total dose of 1 mg is given (initial dose and 4 doses) prn. Usually 0.6-1 mg. If resedation, may repeat after 20 min. Max 1 mg at one time and 3 mg/hr.
➤ *Suspected benzodiazepine overdose—***Adult:** 0.2 mg IV over 30 sec. After 30 sec,

0.3 mg given over 30 sec prn. If poor response, 0.5 mg over 30 sec; repeat 0.5-mg doses prn, at 1-min intervals until total dose of 3 mg. Usually 1-3 mg; rarely, patients may need more doses. Max 5 mg. If resedation, may repeat after 20 min. Max 1 mg at one time and 3 mg/hr.

fluorouracil (5-fluorouracil, 5-FU)
Adrucil, Carac, Efudex, Fluoroplex

Antimetabolite (cell cycle–phase specific, S phase); antineoplastic
PRC: D (injection), X (topical)

Available forms
Cream: 1, 5%; *Injection:* 50 mg/ml; *Topical solution:* 1, 2, 5%

Indications & dosages
➤ *Colon, rectal, breast, stomach, pancreatic CA*—**Adult:** 12 mg/kg IV daily × 4 d; if no toxicity, 6 mg/kg on d 6, 8, 10, and 12; then single wkly maintenance dose of 10-15 mg/kg IV after toxicity subsides. Max single dose 800 mg/d.
➤ *Advanced colorectal CA*—**Adult:** 425 mg/m^2 IV daily × 5 d. Give with 20 mg/m^2 leucovorin IV. Repeat at 4-wk intervals for 2 additional courses; repeat at intervals of 4-5 wk if tolerated.
➤ *Superficial basal cell CA*—**Adult:** Apply cream (5%) or topical solution (5%) bid × 3-6 wk.
➤ *Multiple actinic or solar keratosis of face and anterior scalp*—**Adult:** Wash and dry lesion area; wait 10 min. Apply thin layer to lesions daily for up to 4 wk.

fluoxetine hydrochloride
Prozac, Prozac Weekly, Sarafem

SSRI; antidepressant
PRC: C

Available forms
Capsules: 10, 20, 40 mg; *Capsules (delayed-release):* 90 mg; *Oral solution:* 20 mg/5 ml; *Pulvules:* 10, 20, 40 mg; *Tablets:* 10 mg

Indications & dosages
➤ *Depression (Prozac)*—**Adult:** 20 mg PO q am; increase dose prn. Give doses > 20 mg bid. Max daily dose 80 mg.†,‡
Elderly: 20 mg PO daily q am.†,‡ **Child 8-18 yr:** 10-20 mg P.O. daily. After 1 wk at 10 mg/d, increase dose to 20 mg/d. Lower-weight children should be started at 10 mg/d and dose increased to 20 mg/d after several wk.†,‡
➤ *Maintenance treatment for depression in stabilized patients (Prozac Weekly)*—**Adult:** 90 mg PO once/wk. Initiate once/wk dosing 7 d after last daily dose of Prozac 20 mg.†,‡
➤ *OCD (Prozac)*—**Adult:** 20 mg PO in am; increase dose prn. Give doses > 20 mg bid. Max daily dose 80 mg.†,‡ **Child 7-17 yr:** 10 mg PO daily. After 2 wk, increase dose to 20 mg/d. Dosage range is 20-60 mg/d. Lower-weight children should be increased to 20-30 mg/d after several wk. Max 60 mg daily.†,‡
➤ *Bulimia nervosa (Prozac)*—**Adult:** 60 mg/d PO q am.†,‡
➤ *Short-term treatment of panic disorder (Prozac)*—**Adults:** 10 mg PO daily ×

---

1 wk, then increase dose prn, to 20 mg daily. Max 60 mg daily.

➤ *PMDD (Sarafem)*—**Adult:** 20 mg PO daily continuously or intermittently (starting 14 d before anticipated onset of menstruation through the first full day of menses). Max 80 mg PO daily.†,‡

fluphenazine decanoate
Modecate*, Prolixin Decanoate

fluphenazine enanthate

fluphenazine hydrochloride
Moditen HCl*

Phenothiazine; antipsychotic
PRC: NR

Available forms
decanoate, enanthate *Depot injection:* 25 mg/ml; **hydrochloride** *IM injection:* 2.5 mg/ml; *Tablets:* 1, 2.5, 5, 10 mg

Indications & dosages
➤ *Psychotic disorders*—**Adult:** 0.5-10 mg (HCl) PO daily in divided doses q 6-8 hr; increase to 20 mg prn. Maintenance 1-5 mg PO daily. For IM, give ⅓-½ of PO doses (usual 1.25 mg). Use doses > 10 mg/d cautiously. Or, 12.5-25 mg of long-acting esters (decanoate) IM or SC q 1-6 wk; maintenance 25-100 mg prn. **Elderly:** 1-2.5 mg daily (HCl).

fluticasone propionate (inhalation)
Flovent Inhalation Aerosol, Flovent Rotadisk

Corticosteroid; anti-inflammatory
PRC: C

Available forms
Oral inhalation aerosol: 44, 110, 220 mcg; *Oral inhalation powder:* 50, 100, 250 mcg

Indications & dosages
➤ *Asthma*—*Inhalation aerosol:* **Adult, child ≥ 12 yr:** If previously using bronchodilators only, inhalation dose 88 mcg bid; max 440 mcg bid. Patient previously using inhalation corticosteroids: Inhalation dose 88-220 mcg bid; max 440 mcg bid. Patient previously using PO corticosteroids: Inhalation dose 880 mcg bid. *Rotadisk:* **Adult, child ≥ 12 yr:** Patient previously using bronchodilators only, inhalation dose 100 mcg bid; max 500 mcg bid. Patient previously using inhalation corticosteroids: Inhalation dose 100-250 mcg bid; max 500 mcg bid. Patient previously using PO corticosteroids: Inhalation dose 1,000 mcg bid. **Child 4-11 yr:** Patient previously using bronchodilators only or inhalation corticosteroids, inhalation dose 50 mcg bid; max 100 mcg bid.

fluticasone propionate (nasal)
Flonase

Corticosteroid; topical anti-inflammatory
PRC: C

---

§ Adjust in immunocompromised patients ¶ Adjust in debilitated patients

Available forms
Nasal spray: 50 mcg/metered spray (9-, 16-g bottles)

Indications & dosages
➤ *Nasal symptoms of seasonal and perennial allergic and nonallergic rhinitis*—**Adult:** 2 sprays in each nostril daily or 1 spray bid. Maintenance 1 spray in each nostril daily. Or, for seasonal allergic rhinitis, 2 sprays in each nostril daily prn. **Child ≥ 4 yr:** 1 spray in each nostril daily. May increase to 2 sprays in each nostril daily; then decrease to 1 spray in each nostril daily based on response. Max 2 sprays in each nostril daily.

fluvastatin sodium
Lescol

HMG-CoA reductase inhibitor; antilipemic
PRC: X

Available forms
Capsules: 20, 40 mg; *Tablets (extended-release):* 80 mg

Indications & dosages
➤ *Primary hypercholesterolemia, mixed dyslipidemia*—**Adult:** 20-40 mg PO daily hs or bid; increase prn to max 80 mg/d (in divided doses). Or, 80 mg daily hs (extended-release tablet).

fluvoxamine maleate
Luvox

SSRI; antidepressant
PRC: C

Available forms
Tablets: 25, 50, 100 mg

Indications & dosages
➤ *OCD*—**Adult:** 50 mg PO daily hs; increase in 50-mg increments q 4-7 d prn. Max 300 mg daily. If total daily dose > 100 mg, give in 2 divided doses. **Elderly:** Use a lower initial dose and slower dose adjustment.† **Child 8-17 yr:** 25 mg PO hs. Increase in 25-mg increments q 4 to 7 d until maximum benefit is achieved. Max 200 mg for children 8-11 yr; for children 11-17 yr, max 300 mg. Give total daily doses exceeding 50 mg in two divided doses.†

folic acid
Folvite, Novo-Folacid*

Folic acid derivative; vitamin supplement
PRC: A

Available forms
Injection: 10-ml vials (5 mg/ml with 1.5% benzyl alcohol, 5 mg/ml with 1.5% benzyl alcohol and 0.2% EDTA); *Tablets:* 0.4, 0.8, 1 mg

Indications & dosages
➤ *RDA*—**Man, boy ≥ 11 yr:** 150-200 mcg. **Woman, girl ≥ 11 yr:** 150-180 mcg. **Child 7-10 yr:** 100 mcg. **Child 4-6 yr:** 75 mcg. **Birth-3 yr:** 25-50 mcg. **Pregnant woman:** 400 mcg. **Breast-feeding woman:** 260-280 mcg.
➤ *Megaloblastic or macrocytic anemia*—**Adult, child ≥ 4 yr:** 0.4-1 mg PO, SC, or IM daily. After correction of anemia, proper diet and RDA supplements needed.

Child < 4 yr: Up to 0.3 mg PO, SC, or IM daily. **Pregnant and breast-feeding woman:** 0.8 mg PO, SC, or IM daily.
➤ *Prevention of megaloblastic anemia in pregnancy*—**Adult:** Up to 1 mg PO, SC, or IM daily in pregnancy.

fondaparinux sodium
Arixtra

Inhibitor of activated factor X (Xa); anticoagulant
PRC: B

Available forms
Injection: 2.5 mg/0.5 ml single-dose pre-filled syringe

Indications & dosages
➤ *DVT prevention in patients having hip fracture, hip replacement, or knee replacement surgery*—**Adult:** 2.5 mg SC daily × 5-9 d; max 11 d. Give initial dose after hemostasis is established, 6-8 hr after surgery.

formoterol fumarate inhalation powder
Foradil Aerolizer

Long-acting selective beta$_2$ blocker; bronchodilator
PRC: C

Available forms
Capsules for inhalation: 12 mcg

Indications & dosages
➤ *Prevention and maintenance treatment for bronchospasm in patients with re-* versible obstructive airway disease or nocturnal asthma who usually need treatment with short-acting inhaled beta$_2$-adrenergic agonists—**Adult, child ≥ 5 yr:** One 12-mcg capsule by inhalation via Aerolizer inhaler q 12 hr. Max 1 capsule bid (24 mcg/d). If symptoms are present between doses, use short-acting beta$_2$-adrenergic agonist for immediate relief.
➤ *Prevention of exercise-induced bronchospasm*—**Adult, child ≥ 12 yr:** One 12-mcg cap by inhalation via Aerolizer inhaler at least 15 min before exercise, given occasionally prn. Avoid giving additional doses within 12 hr of 1st dose.
➤ *Maintenance treatment of COPD*—**Adult:** One 12-mcg capsule q 12 hr using the Aerolizer inhaler. Total daily dose of > 24 mcg isn't recommended.

foscarnet sodium (phosphonoformic acid)
Foscavir

Pyrophosphate analogue; antiviral
PRC: C

Available forms
Injection: 24 mg/ml in 250-, 500-ml bottles

Indications & dosages
➤ *CMV retinitis in AIDS patients*—**Adult:** *Induction treatment:* 60 mg/kg IV infusion over 1 hr q 8 hr × 2-3 wk or 90 mg/kg infusion over 1.5-2 hr q 12 hr × 2-3 wk. Then maintenance infusion of 90-120 mg/kg/d over 2 hr.†

---

§ Adjust in immunocompromised patients   ¶ Adjust in debilitated patients

➤ *Mucocutaneous acyclovir-resistant HSV*—**Adult:** 40 mg/kg IV over 1 hr q 8-12 hr × 2-3 wk.†

fosinopril sodium
Monopril

ACE inhibitor; antihypertensive
PRC: C (D, 2nd and 3rd trimesters)

Available forms
Tablets: 10, 20, 40 mg

Indications & dosages
➤ *HTN*—**Adult:** 10 mg PO daily. Adjust based on BP peak and trough levels. Usual dose 20-40 mg; max 80 mg daily, may be divided.
➤ *HF*—**Adult:** 10 mg PO daily. Increase over several wk to max 40 mg PO daily.

fosphenytoin sodium
Cerebyx

Hydantoin derivative; anticonvulsant
PRC: D

Available forms
Injection: 2 ml (150 mg fosphenytoin sodium = 100 mg phenytoin sodium), 10 ml (750 mg fosphenytoin sodium = 500 mg phenytoin sodium)

Indications & dosages
➤ *Status epilepticus*—**Adult:** 15-20 mg phenytoin sodium equivalent (PE)/kg IV at 100-150 mg PE/min as loading dose; then 4-6 mg PE/kg/d IV as maintenance. (Phenytoin may be used instead.)

➤ *Seizures during neurosurgery*—**Adult:** Loading dose 10-20 mg PE/kg IM or IV at rate ≤ 150 mg PE/min. Maintenance 4-6 mg PE/kg/d IV.
➤ *Short-term substitution for PO phenytoin*—**Adult:** Same total daily dose equivalent as PO phenytoin sodium treatment in 1 dose daily IM or IV at ≤ 150 mg PE/min. May require more frequent dosing.

frovatriptan succinate
Frova

5-HT₁ receptor agonist; antimigraine drug
PRC: C

Available forms
Tablets: 2.5 mg

Indications & dosages
➤ *Migraine*—**Adult:** 2.5 mg PO. May repeat dose in ≥ 2 hr if migraine returns after initial dose.

fulvestrant
Faslodex

Estrogen receptor antagonist; antineoplastic
PRC: D

Available forms
Injection: 50 mg/ml in 2.5-ml and 5-ml prefilled syringes

Indications & dosages
➤ *Hormone-receptor–positive metastatic breast CA in postmenopausal women with disease progression following anti-*

---

estrogen therapy—**Adult:** 250 mg by slow IM injection into buttock q month.

furosemide
Apo-Furosemide*, Lasix, Novosemide*

Loop diuretic; diuretic, antihypertensive
PRC: C

Available forms
Injection: 10 mg/ml; *Oral solution:* 10 mg/ml, 40 mg/5 ml; *Tablets:* 20, 40, 80 mg

Indications & dosages
➤ *Pulmonary edema*—**Adult:** 40 mg IV over 1-2 min; then 80 mg IV in 1-1½ hr prn.
➤ *Edema*—**Adult:** 20-80 mg PO daily in am, 2nd dose in 6-8 hr; adjust up to 600 mg daily prn. Or, 20-40 mg IM or IV; increase by 20 mg q 2 hr prn. Give IV dose slowly over 1-2 min. **Infant, child:** 2 mg/kg PO daily; increase by 1-2 mg/kg in 6-8 hr prn; adjust to 6 mg/kg/d prn.
➤ *HTN*—**Adult:** 40 mg PO bid. Adjust dose prn.

gabapentin
Neurontin

1-Aminomethyl cyclohexonacetic acid; anticonvulsant
PRC: C

Available forms
Capsules: 100, 300, 400 mg; *Solution:* 250 mg/5 ml; *Tablets:* 600, 800 mg

Indications & dosages
➤ *Partial seizures*—**Adult:** 300 mg PO hs on d 1; 300 mg PO bid d 2; then 300 mg PO tid d 3. Increase prn to 1,800 mg/d in 3 divided doses. Max 3,600 mg/d.†
➤ *Adjunctive treatment to control partial seizures*—**Child 3-12 yr:** 10-15 mg/kg/d PO in 3 divided doses to start, adjusting over 3 d to reach effective dosages. **Effective dosage, child 5-12 yr:** 25 to 35 mg/kg/d PO in 2 divided doses. **Effective dosage, child 3-4 yr:** 40 mg/kg/d PO in 2 divided doses.†
➤ *Postherpetic neuralgia*—**Adult:** 300 mg PO on d 1, then 300 mg bid on d 2; 300 mg tid on d 3. Max 1,800 mg daily in 3 divided doses.†

galantamine hydrobromide
Reminyl

Reversible, competitive acetylcholinesterase inhibitor; cholinomimetic
PRC: B

Available forms
Oral solution: 4 mg/ml; *Tablets:* 4, 8, 12 mg

Indications & dosages
➤ *Mild to moderate dementia of Alzheimer's type*—**Adult:** Initially, 4 mg bid, preferably with am and pm meal. If dose is well tolerated after minimum of 4 wk of therapy, increase to 8 mg bid. A further increase to 12 mg bid may be attempted only after ≥ 4 wk at previous dose. Recommended range, 16-24 mg/d in 2 divided doses.†,‡

---

§ Adjust in immunocompromised patients   ¶ Adjust in debilitated patients

ganciclovir
Cytovene

Synthetic nucleoside; antiviral
PRC: C

Available forms
Capsules: 250, 500 mg; *Injection:* 500 mg/vial

Indications & dosages
➤ *CMV retinitis in immunocompromised patients and AIDS patients*—**Adult:** 5 mg/kg IV q 12 hr × 14-21 d; maintenance 5 mg/kg IV daily × 7 d/wk, or 6 mg/kg/d × 5 d/wk. Or, 1,000 mg PO tid with food; or 500 mg PO q 3 hr while awake (6 times/d).†
➤ *Prevent CMV in HIV infection*—**Adult:** 1,000 mg PO tid with food.†
➤ *Prevent CMV in transplant recipients*—**Adult:** 5 mg/kg IV q 12 hr × 7-14 d, then 5 mg/kg/d × 7 d/wk; or 6 mg/kg/d × 5 d/wk.†

gatifloxacin
Tequin

Fluoroquinolone; antibiotic
PRC: C

Available forms
Injection: 200 mg/20-ml vial, 400 mg/40-ml vial; 200 mg/100 ml D₅W, 400 mg/200 ml D₅W; *Tablets:* 200, 400 mg

Indications & dosages
➤ *Complicated UTI, pyelonephritis*—**Adult:** 400 mg IV or PO daily × 7-10 d.†

➤ *Sinusitis*—**Adult:** 400 mg IV or PO daily × 10 d.†
➤ *Community-acquired pneumonia*—**Adult:** 400 mg IV or PO daily × 7-14 d.†
➤ *Urethral gonorrhea in man; cervical gonorrhea or rectal infection in woman from* Neisseria gonorrhoeae—**Adult:** 400 mg PO × 1 dose.†
➤ *Uncomplicated UTI*—**Adult:** 400 mg IV or PO × 1 dose, or 200 mg IV or PO daily × 3 d.†
➤ *Acute bacterial exacerbation of chronic bronchitis from* Streptococcus pneumoniae, Haemophilus influenzae, H. parainfluenzae, Moraxella catarrhalis, *or* Staphylococcus aureus—**Adult:** 400 mg IV or PO daily × 5 d.†
➤ *Uncomplicated skin and skin-structure infections from* Staphylococcus aureus (methicillin-susceptible strains only) *or* Streptococcus pyogenes—**Adult:** 400 mg IV or PO daily × 7-10 d.†

gemfibrozil
Lopid

Fibric acid derivative; antilipemic
PRC: C

Available forms
Tablets: 600 mg

Indications & dosages
➤ *Types IV and V hyperlipidemia, CAD risk reduction in type IIb hyperlipidemia*—**Adult:** 1,200 mg PO daily in 2 divided doses, 30 min ac in am and pm.

---

gentamicin sulfate (systemic)

Cidomycin*, Garamycin, Gentamicin Sulfate, Jenamicin

Aminoglycoside; antibiotic
PRC: NR

Available forms

Injection: 40 mg/ml (adult), 10 mg/ml (pediatric), 2 mg/ml (intrathecal); *IV infusion (premixed):* 40, 60, 70, 80, 90, 100, 120 mg in NSS

Indications & dosages

➤ *Serious infection*—**Adult:** 3 mg/kg/d in divided doses IM or IV infusion q 8 hr. Life-threatening infection, up to 5 mg/kg/d in 3-4 divided doses; reduce to 3 mg/kg/d ASAP. **Child:** 6-7.5 mg/kg/d in divided doses q 8 hr IM or IV infusion. **Neonate > 1 wk, infant:** 7.5 mg/kg/d in divided doses q 8 hr.
➤ *Meningitis*—**Adult:** Systemic treatment as above; or 4-8 mg intrathecally daily. **Child, infant > 3 mo:** Systemic treatment as above; or 1-2 mg intrathecally daily.
➤ *Endocarditis prophylaxis for GI, GU procedure, or surgery*—**Adult:** 1.5 mg/kg IM or IV 30 min before procedure or surgery. Max 80 mg. **Child:** 2 mg/kg IM or IV 30 min before procedure or surgery. Max 80 mg. After 8 hr, ½ initial dose.

glimepiride

Amaryl

Sulfonylurea; antidiabetic
PRC: C

Available forms

Tablets: 1, 2, 4 mg

Indications & dosages

➤ *Type 2 DM*—**Adult:** 1-2 mg PO daily with 1st main meal of d; maintenance 1-4 mg PO daily. After reaching 2 mg, increase dose up to 2 mg q 1-2 wk, based on glucose level. Max 8 mg/d.†
➤ *Adjunct to insulin therapy in type 2 DM*—**Adult:** 8 mg PO daily with 1st main meal of d; use with low-dose insulin.†
➤ *Adjunct to metformin in type 2 DM*—**Adult:** 8 mg PO daily with 1st main meal of d with metformin. Adjust doses prn.†

glipizide

Glucotrol, Glucotrol XL

Sulfonylurea; antidiabetic
PRC: C

Available forms

Tablets: 5, 10 mg; *Tablets (extended-release):* 5, 10 mg

Indications & dosages

➤ *Type 2 DM*—**Adult:** 5 mg PO 30 min before breakfast. Maintenance 10-15 mg; max 40 mg daily. Daily doses above 15 mg can be divided bid. *Extended-release:* 5 mg PO daily given with breakfast. Adjust in 5-mg increments q 3 mo. Max 20 mg daily.‡,¶
➤ *Replace insulin treatment*—**Adult:** Insulin dosage > 20 units daily; start at 5 mg PO daily plus 50% of insulin. If insulin dose < 20 units, stop insulin when starting glipizide.‡,¶

---

§ Adjust in immunocompromised patients　　　　¶ Adjust in debilitated patients

glipizide and metformin hydrochloride
Metaglip

Sulfonylurea and biguanide; antidiabetic
PRC: C

Available forms
Tablets: 2.5 mg glipizide and 250 mg metformin hydrochloride; 2.5 mg glipizide and 500 mg metformin; 5 mg glipizide and 500 mg metformin

Indications & dosages
➤ *Type 2 DM with diet and exercise—*
Adult: Initially 2.5 mg/250 mg PO daily with a meal. Patients with fasting glucose 280 to 320 mg/dl, start with 2.5 mg/ 500 mg PO bid. May increase dose by one tablet daily q 2 wk. Max 10 mg/ 1,000 mg or 10 mg/2,000 mg daily in divided doses.
➤ *Type 2 DM when diet, exercise, and treatment with sulfonylurea or metformin fail—***Adult:** Initially 2.5 mg/500 mg or 5 mg/500 mg PO bid with am and pm meals. Increase by ≤ 5 mg/500 mg. Max 20 mg/2,000 mg daily.

glucagon

Antihypoglycemic; antidiabetic, diagnostic aid
PRC: B

Available forms
Powder for injection: 1-mg (1-units), 10-mg (10-units) vial

Indications & dosages
➤ *Hypoglycemia—***Adult, child > 20 kg:** 1 mg SC, IM, or IV; may repeat in 15 min prn. In deep coma, also give glucose 10- 50% IV. **Child ≤ 20 kg:** 0.5 mg SC, IM, or IV. In deep coma, also give glucose 10- 50% IV. May repeat in 15 min prn.
➤ *Diagnostic aid for radiologic exam—*
Adult: 0.25-2 mg IV or IM before radiologic procedure.

glyburide (glibenclamide)
DiaBeta, Euglucon*, Glynase PresTab, Micronase

Sulfonylurea; antidiabetic
PRC: C

Available forms
Tablets: 1.25, 2.5, 5 mg; *Tablets (micronized):* 1.5, 3, 4.5, 6 mg

Indications & dosages
➤ *Type 2 DM—***Adult:** 2.5-5 mg regular tablet PO daily with breakfast. Maintenance 1.25-20 mg daily in 1 dose or divided doses or may use micronized preparation. Initially 1.5-3 mg daily. In sensitive patients, 0.75 mg daily. Maintenance 0.75-12 mg/d. Patients receiving > 6 mg/d, use bid. In debilitated, malnourished, or elderly patients or those with adrenal or pituitary insufficiency, 1.25 mg/d.
➤ *Replace insulin treatment—***Adult:** Insulin dose > 40 units/d, 5 mg/d plus 50% of insulin dose; if < 20 units/d, 2.5- 5 mg/d; if 20-40 units/d, 5 mg/d. In all patients, substitute glyburide and stop

---

*Canadian   † Adjust in renal impairment   ‡ Adjust in liver impairment

insulin. For micronized tablet, if insulin dose > 40 units/d, 3 mg PO with 50% reduction in insulin; if 20-40 units/d, 3 mg PO daily; if < 20 units/d, 1.5-3 mg/d. Adjust dose in malnourished or elderly patients or those with adrenal or pituitary insufficiency.¶

granisetron hydrochloride
Kytril

Selective 5-hydroxy-tryptamine receptor antagonist; antiemetic, antinauseant
PRC: B

Available forms
Injection: 1 mg/ml; *Oral solution:* 1 mg/ 5 ml; *Tablets:* 1 mg

Indications & dosages
➤ *Prevent nausea, vomiting with emetogenic CA chemo*—**Adult, child ≥ 2:** 10 mcg/kg IV undiluted by direct injection over 30 sec, or diluted and infused over 5 min. Begin administration within 30 min of chemo initiation. Or, for adults, 1 mg PO up to 1 hr before chemo and repeated 12 hr later. Or, for adults, 2 mg PO daily given ≤ 1 hr before chemo.
➤ *Postop nausea and vomiting*—**Adult:** 1 mg IV undiluted over 30 sec. For prevention, give before anesthesia induction or immediately before reversal.
➤ *Prevent nausea, vomiting with radiation*—**Adult:** 2 mg PO daily within 1 hr of radiation.

griseofulvin microsize
Fulvicin-U/F, Grifulvin V, Grisactin, Grisovin-FP

griseofulvin ultramicrosize
Fulvicin P/G, Grisactin Ultra, Gris-PEG

PCN antibiotic; antifungal
PRC: C

Available forms
microsize *Capsules:* 250 mg; *Oral suspension:* 125 mg/5 ml; *Tablets:* 250, 500 mg; **ultramicrosize** *Tablets:* 125, 165, 250, 330 mg

Indications & dosages
➤ *Ringworm of skin, hair, nails*—**Adult:** 500 mg (microsize) PO daily in 1 dose or in divided doses. Severe infection, up to 1 g/d. Or, 330-375 mg (ultramicrosize) PO daily in 1 dose or in divided doses. **Child > 2 yr:** 125-250 mg (microsize) PO daily. Or, 7.3 mg/kg (ultramicrosize) PO daily for child 13.1-22.7 kg; or, 250-500 mg (microsize) PO daily for child > 22.7 kg.
➤ *Tinea pedis, tinea unguium*—**Adult:** 0.75-1 g (microsize) PO daily. Or, 660-750 mg (ultramicrosize) PO daily in divided doses. **Child > 2 yr:** 125-250 mg (microsize) PO daily. Or, 7.3 mg/kg (ultramicrosize) PO daily for child 13.1-22.7 kg; or, 250-500 mg (microsize) PO daily for child > 22.7 kg.

---

§ Adjust in immunocompromised patients   ¶ Adjust in debilitated patients

guaifenesin (glyceryl guaiacolate)
Anti-Tuss, Duratuss G, Glytuss, Halotussin, Humibid L.A., Mucinex, Robitussin

Propanediol derivative; expectorant
PRC: C

Available forms
Capsules: 200 mg; *Solution:* 100, 200 mg/ 5 ml; *Tablets:* 100, 200 mg; *Tablets (extended-release):* 600, 1,200 mg

Indications & dosages
➤ *Expectorant*—**Adult, child ≥ 12 yr:** 100-400 mg PO q 4 hr, max 2.4 g/d; or, 600-1,200 mg extended-release tablets q 12 hr, max 2,400 mg/d. **Child 6-12 yr:** 100-200 mg PO q 4 hr, max 1,200 mg/d. **Child 2-6 yr:** 50-100 mg PO q 4 hr, max 600 mg/d.

haloperidol
Apo-Haloperidol*, Haldol, Novo-Peridol*, Peridol*

haloperidol decanoate
Haldol Decanoate, Haldol LA*

haloperidol lactate
Haldol

Butyrophenone; antipsychotic
PRC: C

Available forms
haloperidol *Tablets:* 0.5, 1, 2, 5, 10, 20 mg; **decanoate** *Injection:* 50, 100 mg/ ml; **lactate** *Injection:* 5 mg/ml; *Oral concentrate:* 2 mg/ml

Indications & dosages
➤ *Psychotic disorders*—**Adult, child ≥ 12 yr:** 0.5-5 mg PO bid or tid; or 2-5 mg IM q 4-8 hr. Max 100 mg PO daily. **Child 3-11 yr:** 0.05-0.15 mg/kg PO daily in 2-3 divided doses.
➤ *Chronic psychosis*—**Adult:** 50-100 mg IM decanoate q 4 wk.¶
➤ *Nonpsychotic behavior disorders*— **Child 3-12 yr:** 0.05 mg/kg PO daily. Max 6 mg/d.

heparin sodium
Hepalean*

Anticoagulant; anticoagulant, antithrombotic
PRC: C

Available forms
sodium *Carpuject:* 5,000 units/ml; *Disposable syringes:* 1,000, 2,500, 10,000, 15,000, 20,000, 40,000 units/ml; *Flush (disposable syringes, vials):* 10, 100 units/ ml; *Premixed IV solution:* 1,000 units in 500 ml NSS; 2,000 units in 1,000 ml NSS; 12,500, 25,000 units in 250 ml ½ NSS; 25,000 units in 500 ml ½ NSS; 10,000 units in 100 ml D₅W; 12,500, 25,000 units in 250 ml D₅W; 20,000, 25,000 units in 500 ml D₅W; *Unit-dose vials:* 1,000, 5,000, 10,000, 20,000, 40,000 units/ml; *Vials:* 1,000, 2,000, 2,500, 5,000, 7,500, 10,000, 20,000, 40,000 units/ml

Indications & dosages

➤ *Full-dose IV infusion treatment for DVT, MI, PE*—**Adult:** 5,000 units IV bolus; then 750-1,500 units/hr IV infusion pump. Adjust hourly rate 8 hr after bolus dose, based on PTT. **Child:** 50 units/kg IV; then 25 units/kg/hr or 20,000 units/m² daily by IV infusion pump. Adjust dose based on PTT.

➤ *Full-dose SC treatment for DVT, MI, PE*—**Adult:** 5,000 units IV bolus and 10,000-20,000 units in concentrated solution SC; then 8,000-10,000 units SC q 8 hr or 15,000-20,000 units in concentrated solution q 12 hr.

➤ *Fixed low-dose treatment for venous thrombosis, postop DVT, PE, atrial fibrillation with embolism, embolism prevention*—**Adult:** 5,000 units SC q 12 hr. In surgery patients, give 1st dose 2 hr before surgery, then 5,000 units SC q 8-12 hr × 5-7 d or until patient can walk.

➤ *Consumptive coagulopathy (such as disseminated intravascular coagulation)*—**Adult:** 50-100 units/kg IV bolus or continuous IV infusion q 4 hr. **Child:** 25-50 units/kg IV bolus or continuous IV infusion q 4 hr. If no improvement within 4-8 hr, stop treatment.

hydralazine hydrochloride
Apresoline, Novo-Hylazin*

Peripheral vasodilator; antihypertensive
PRC: C

Available forms
Injection: 20 mg/ml; *Tablets:* 10, 25, 50, 100 mg

Indications & dosages

➤ *HTN (PO), severe HTN (parenteral)*—**Adult:** PO: 10 mg qid; increase to 50 mg qid. Max 200 mg/d (300-400 mg/d in some patients). IV: 10-20 mg repeated prn; switch to PO ASAP. IM: 20-40 mg repeated prn; switch to PO ASAP. **Child:** PO: 0.75 mg/kg/d in 4 divided doses; increase over 3-4 wk. Max 7.5 mg/kg or 200 mg daily. IV or IM: 1.7-3.5 mg/kg/d or 50-100 mg/m²/d in 4-6 divided doses. Initial parenteral dose ≤ 20 mg.

hydrochlorothiazide (HCTZ)
Apo-Hydro*, Aquazide-H, Esidrix, HydroDIURIL, Oretic

Thiazide diuretic; diuretic, antihypertensive
PRC: B

Available forms
Capsules: 12.5 mg; *Oral solution:* 50 mg/5 ml; *Tablets:* 25, 50, 100 mg

Indications & dosages

➤ *Edema*—**Adult:** 25-100 mg PO daily or intermittently.

➤ *HTN*—**Adult:** 12.5-50 mg PO daily. Increase or decrease dose based on BP. **Child 2-12 yr:** 2.2 mg/kg or 60 mg/m² daily in 2 divided doses. Usual, 37.5-100 mg/d. **Child 6 mo-2 yr:** 2.2 mg/kg or 60 mg/m² daily in 2 divided doses. Usual, 12.5-37.5 mg/d. **Child < 6 mo:** Max 3.3 mg/kg daily in 2 divided doses.

hydrocortisone (systemic)
Cortef, Hydrocortone

hydrocortisone acetate
Cortifoam, Hydrocortone Acetate

hydrocortisone sodium phosphate
Hydrocortone Phosphate

hydrocortisone sodium succinate
A-hydroCort, Solu-Cortef

Glucocorticoid, mineralocorticoid; adrenocorticoid replacement
PRC: C

Available forms
hydrocortisone *Enema:* 100 mg/60 ml; *Tablets:* 5, 10, 20 mg; **acetate** *Enema:* 10% aerosol foam (90 mg/application); *Injection:* 25 mg/ml, 50 mg/ml suspension; **sodium phosphate** *Injection:* 50 mg/ml solution; **sodium succinate** *Injection:* 100, 250, 500, 1,000 mg/vial

Indications & dosages
➤ *Severe inflammation, adrenal insufficiency*—**Adult:** 5-30 mg PO bid-qid (up to 80 mg qid). Or, 100-500 mg succinate IM or IV, then 50-100 mg IM; or, 15-240 mg phosphate IM or IV daily in divided doses q 12 hr; or 5-75 mg acetate into joints or soft tissue. Local anesthetics often injected with dose.
➤ *Shock*—**Adult:** 50 mg/kg succinate IV repeated in 4 hr. Repeat q 24 hr prn. Or, 100-500 mg to 2 g q 2-6 hr; continue until patient is stabilized. **Child:** phosphate

(IM) or succinate (IM or IV) 0.16-1 mg/kg or 6-30 mg/m² daily or bid.

hydrocortisone (topical)
Acticort, CaldeCORT, Cortef, Cortizone 5

hydrocortisone acetate
CortaGel, Cortaid, Cortamed*, Hydrocortisone Acetate

hydrocortisone butyrate
Locoid

hydrocortisone valerate
Westcort

Glucocorticoid; topical adrenocorticoid
PRC: C

Available forms
hydrocortisone (topical) *Aerosol:* 0.5%, 1%; *Cream:* 0.25%, 0.5%, 1%, 2.5%; *Enema:* 100 mg/60 ml; *Gel:* 0.5%, 1%; *Lotion:* 0.125%, 0.25%, 0.5%, 1%, 2%, 2.5%; *Ointment:* 0.5%, 1%, 2.5%; *Pledgets:* 0.5%, 1%; *Rectal cream:* 1%; *Stick roll-on:* 1%; *Suppository:* 25 mg; *Topical solution:* 0.5%, 1%, 2.5%; **acetate** *Cream, ointment:* 0.5%, 1%; *Lotion:* 0.5%; *Paste:* 0.5%; *Rectal foam:* 90 mg/application; *Solution:* 1%; *Suppository:* 10, 25 mg; **butyrate** *Cream, ointment, solution:* 0.1%; **valerate** *Cream, ointment:* 0.2%

Indications & dosages
➤ *Dermatitis, topical management of seborrheic scalp dermatitis*—**Adult, child:** Clean area; apply cream, gel, lotion, ointment, or topical solution sparingly once

---

*Canadian   † Adjust in renal impairment   ‡ Adjust in liver impairment

daily to qid. Spray aerosol on affected area once daily to qid for acute phase; then reduce to 1-3 times/wk prn.
➤ *Inflammation in proctitis*—**Adult:** 1 applicator rectal foam PR daily or bid × 2-3 wk; then q other d prn.

hydromorphone hydrochloride (dihydromorphinone hydrochloride)
Dilaudid, Dilaudid-HP

Opioid; analgesic, antitussive
PRC: C; CSS: II

Available forms
Injection: 1, 2, 4, 10 mg/ml; *Liq:* 5 mg/5 ml; *Suppository:* 3 mg; *Tablets:* 1, 2, 3, 4, 8 mg

Indications & dosages
➤ *Pain*—**Adult:** 2-10 mg PO q 3-6 hr prn or around-the-clock. Or, 2-4 mg IM, SC, or IV (over ≥ 3-5 min) q 4-6 hr prn or around-the-clock; or, 3 mg PR hs prn or around-the-clock. (Give 1-14 mg Dilaudid-HP SC or IM q 4-6 hr.)
➤ *Cough*—**Adult, adolescent > 12 yr:** 1 mg PO q 3-4 hr prn. **Child 6-12 yr:** 0.5 mg PO q 3-4 hr prn.

hydroxyzine hydrochloride
Apo-Hydroxyzine*, Atarax, Hyzine-50, Multipax*, Vistaril, Vistazine 50

hydroxyzine pamoate
Vistaril

Antihistamine (piperazine derivative); anxiolytic, sedative, antipruritic, antiemetic, antispasmodic
PRC: C

Available forms
hydrochloride *Capsules*:* 10, 25, 50 mg; *Injection:* 25, 50 mg/ml; *Syrup:* 10 mg/5 ml; *Tablets:* 10, 25, 50, 100 mg; **pamoate** *Capsules:* 25, 50, 100 mg; *Oral suspension:* 25 mg/5 ml

Indications & dosages
➤ *Anxiety, tension, hyperkinesias*—**Adult:** 50-100 mg PO qid. **Child ≥ 6 yr:** 50-100 mg PO daily in divided doses. **Child < 6 yr:** 50 mg PO daily in divided doses.
➤ *Preop, postop adjunctive sedation; vomiting; asthma*—**Adult:** 25-100 mg IM q 4-6 hr. **Child:** 1.1 mg/kg IM q 4-6 hr.
➤ *Pruritus from allergies*—**Adult:** 25 mg PO tid or qid. **Child ≥ 6 yr:** 50-100 mg PO daily in divided doses. **Child < 6 yr:** 50 mg PO daily in divided doses.

ibuprofen
Advil, Children's Advil, Children's Motrin, Motrin, Motrin IB, Motrin-IB Caplets, Nuprin, Nuprin Caplets, Pedia-Profen

NSAID; nonopioid analgesic, antipyretic, anti-inflammatory
PRC: B

Available forms
Tablets: 100, 200, 400, 600, 800 mg; *Tablets (chewable):* 50, 100 mg; *Oral suspension:* 100 mg/2.5 ml, 100 mg/5 ml; *Oral drops:* 40 mg/ml

Indications & dosages

➤ *RA, OA, arthritis*—**Adult:** 300-800 mg PO tid or qid. Max 3.2 g/d.

➤ *Pain, dysmenorrhea*—**Adult:** 400 mg PO q 4-6 hr prn.

➤ *Fever*—**Adult:** 200-400 mg PO q 4-6 hr. Don't exceed 1.2 g daily or give > 3 d. **Child 6 mo-12 yr:** If temp < 39° C, 5 mg/kg PO q 6-8 hr. Higher temps, 10 mg/kg q 6-8 hr. Max 40 mg/kg/d.

➤ *Juvenile arthritis*—**Child:** 30-70 mg/kg/d in 3-4 divided doses.

imatinib mesylate
Gleevec

Protein-tyrosine kinase inhibitor; antineoplastic
PRC: D

Available forms

Capsules: 50, 100 mg; *Tablets:* 100, 400 mg

Indications & dosages

➤ *Philadelphia chromosome-positive chronic myeloid leukemia (CML) in newly diagnosed patients; Philadelphia chromosome-positive CML in blast crisis, accelerated phase, or chronic phase after failure of interferon-alpha treatment*—**Adult:** For chronic-phase CML, 400 mg PO daily as single dose with a meal and large glass of H$_2$O. May increase dose to 600 mg PO daily.‡،§ For accelerated-phase CML or blast crisis, 600 mg PO daily as single dose with a meal and large glass of H$_2$O. May increase to 400 mg PO bid. Continue treatment as long as patient benefits.‡،§

➤ *Kit (CD117)-positive unresectable or metastatic malignant GI stromal tumor*—**Adult:** 400 or 600 mg PO daily.‡،§

imipenem and cilastatin
Primaxin IM, Primaxin IV

Carbapenem (thienamycin class) beta-lactam antibiotic; antibiotic
PRC: C

Available forms

Powder for injection: 250, 500, 750 mg

Indications & dosages

➤ *Serious lower respiratory, urinary tract, intra-abdominal, GYN, bone, joint, skin, soft-tissue infection; bacterial septicemia and endocarditis*—**Adult, child ≥ 40 kg:** 250 mg-1 g by IV infusion q 6-8 hr. Max 50 mg/kg/d or 4 g/d, whichever is less. Or, 500-750 mg IM q 12 hr. Don't use IM for septicemia or endocarditis. Max 1,500 mg/d. **Child < 40 kg:** 60 mg/kg IV daily in divided doses. **Infant < 36 wk gestational age:** 20 mg/kg IV q 12 hr.†

imipramine hydrochloride
Apo-Imipramine*, Imipril*, Norfranil, Tipramine, Tofranil

imipramine pamoate
Tofranil-PM

Dibenzazepine-derivative TCA; antidepressant
PRC: B

---

*Canadian   † Adjust in renal impairment   ‡ Adjust in liver impairment

Available forms
hydrochloride *Tablets:* 10, 25, 50 mg;
pamoate *Capsules:* 75, 100, 125, 150 mg

Indications & dosages
➤ *Depression*—**Adult:** 75-100 mg PO daily in divided doses; increase in 25-50 mg increments. Max (outpatients) 200 mg/d; max (inpatients) 300 mg/d. Entire dose may be given hs. **Elderly, child ≥ 12 yr:** 30-40 mg daily. Max 100 mg/d.
➤ *Childhood enuresis*—**Child ≥ 6 yr:** 25 mg PO 1 hr before hs. If no response within 1 wk, increase to 50 mg if child < 12 yr; 75 mg if child ≥ 12 yr. Max 2.5 mg/kg/d.

inamrinone lactate

Bipyridine derivative; inotropic, vasodilator
PRC: C

Available forms
Injection: 5 mg/ml

Indications & dosages
➤ *Short-term management of HF*—
Adult: Initially, 0.75 mg/kg IV bolus over 2-3 min; then begin maintenance infusion of 5-10 mcg/kg/min. Additional bolus of 0.75 mg/kg may be given 30 min after treatment starts. Max 10 mg/kg/d.

indapamide
Lozide*, Lozol

Thiazide-like diuretic; diuretic, antihypertensive
PRC: B

Available forms
Tablets: 1.25, 2.5 mg

Indications & dosages
➤ *Edema*—**Adult:** 2.5 mg PO daily in am. Increase to 5 mg/d after 1 wk prn.
➤ *HTN*—**Adult:** 1.25 mg PO daily in am. Increase to 2.5 mg/d after 4 wk prn. Increase to 5 mg/d after 4 more wk prn.

indinavir sulfate
Crixivan

HIV protease inhibitor; antiviral
PRC: C

Available forms
Capsules: 100, 200, 333, 400 mg

Indications & dosages
➤ *HIV infection*—**Adult:** 800 mg PO q 8 hr.‡

indomethacin
Apo-Indomethacin*, Indochron ER, Indocid SR*, Indocin, Indocin SR, Novo-Methacin*

NSAID; nonopioid analgesic, antipyretic, anti-inflammatory
PRC: NR

Available forms
Capsules: 25, 50 mg; *Capsules (sustained-release):* 75 mg; *Oral suspension:* 25 mg/ 5 ml; *Suppository:* 50 mg

Indications & dosages
➤ *RA, OA, ankylosing spondylitis*—**Adult:** 25 mg PO or PR bid or tid with food or

---

§ Adjust in immunocompromised patients　　　¶ Adjust in debilitated patients

antacids; increase daily dose 25 or 50 mg q 7 d. Max 200 mg daily. Or, sustained-release 75 mg PO in am or hs; then 75 mg bid prn.

➤ *Gouty arthritis*—**Adult:** 50 mg PO tid. Reduce ASAP; then stop.

➤ *Shoulder bursitis or tendinitis*—**Adult:** 75-150 mg PO daily in divided doses tid or qid × 7-14 d.

insulin injection (regular insulin, crystalline zinc insulin)
Humulin R, Iletin II Regular, Novolin R, Purified Pork

insulin (lispro)
Humalog

isophane insulin suspension (NPH)
Humulin N, Novolin N, NPH Insulin

isophane insulin suspension with insulin injection
Humulin 50/50, Humulin 70/30, Novolin 70/30

insulin zinc suspension (lente)
Humulin L, Lente Insulin, Novolin L

insulin zinc suspension, extended (ultralente)
Humulin U, Ultralente Insulin

insulin aspart
NovoLog

insulin glargine
Lantus

Pancreatic hormone; antidiabetic
PRC: B (C, insulin glargine and aspart)

Available forms
Injection: range 100-500 units/ml; human, pork sources; vials to cartridge systems; slow to fast acting

Indications & dosages
➤ *Diabetic ketoacidosis (regular insulin)*—**Adult:** 0.33 units/kg IV bolus; then 0.1 units/kg/hr by continuous infusion. Continue infusion until glucose level 250 mg/dl; then start SC insulin. Or, 50-100 units IV and 50-100 units SC immediately; then additional doses q 2-6 hr based on glucose level. **Child:** 0.1 units/kg IV bolus, then 0.1 units/kg/hr by continuous infusion until glucose level 250 mg/dl; then start SC insulin. Or, 1-2 units/kg in 2 divided doses, 1 IV and 1 SC; then 0.5-1 units/kg IV q 1-2 hr based on glucose level.

➤ *Types 1, 2 DM*—**Adult, child:** Adjust based on glucose level.

➤ *DM (NovoLog)*—**Adult:** Individualize dose; adjust based on glucose level. Give SC within 5-10 min ac.

➤ *Patient needing long-acting insulin (Lantus) who is adult or child with Type 1 DM or adult with Type 2 DM*—**Adult, child ≥ 6 yr:** Individualize dose; give SC daily.

---

irbesartan 79

➤ *Types 1, 2 DM in patient needing long-acting insulin (Lispro)—***Adult, child > 3 yr:** Individualize dose. Inject SC within 15 min ac or immediately afterward.

ipecac syrup
Ipecac Syrup

Alkaloid emetic; emetic
PRC: C

Available forms
Syrup: 70 mg powdered ipecac/ml (contains glycerin 10% and alcohol 1-2.5%)

Indications & dosages
➤ *Induce vomiting in poisoning—***Adult, child ≥ 12 yr:** 30 ml PO; then 200-300 ml H_2O. **Child 1-11 yr:** 15 ml PO; then 240-480 ml H_2O. **Child < 1 yr:** 5-10 ml PO; then 120-240 ml H_2O. Repeat dose in patients > 1 yr if no vomiting within 20 min. If no vomiting within 30-35 min after 2nd dose, perform gastric lavage.

ipratropium bromide
Atrovent

Anticholinergic; bronchodilator
PRC: B

Available forms
Inhalation: 18 mcg/metered dose; *Nasal spray:* 0.03% (21 mcg/metered dose), 0.06% (42 mcg/metered dose); *Solution (for inhalation):* 0.02% (500 mcg/vial)

Indications & dosages
➤ *Bronchospasm in COPD—***Adult, child > 12 yr:** 1-2 inhalations qid. Max 12 in-halations/24 hr. Or, inhalation solution 500 mcg dissolved in NSS via nebulizer q 6-8 hr.
➤ *Rhinorrhea from allergic and non-allergic perennial rhinitis (0.3% nasal spray)—***Adult, child ≥ 6 yr:** 2 sprays (42 mcg) per nostril bid or tid.
➤ *Rhinorrhea from common cold (0.6% nasal spray)—***Adult, child ≥ 12 yr:** 2 sprays (84 mcg) per nostril tid or qid. **Child 5-11 yr:** 2 sprays (84 mcg) per nostril tid.
➤ *Rhinorrhea associated with seasonal allergic rhinitis (0.06% nasal spray)—***Adult, child ≥ 5 yr:** 2 sprays (84 mcg) per nostril qid.

irbesartan
Avapro

Angiotensin II receptor antagonist; antihypertensive
PRC: C (D, 2nd and 3rd trimesters)

Available forms
Tablet: 75, 150, 300 mg

Indications & dosages
➤ *HTN—***Adult, child ≥ 13 yr:** 150 mg PO daily; increase to max 300 mg daily prn. Decrease dose in volume- and salt-depleted patients. **Child 6-12 yr:** 75 mg PO daily; increase to max 150 mg daily prn.
➤ *Nephropathy in type 2 DM—***Adult:** 300 mg PO daily.

§ Adjust in immunocompromised patients ¶ Adjust in debilitated patients

isoniazid (isonicotinic acid hydrazide, INH)
Isotamine*, Laniazid, Nydrazid, PMS-Isoniazid*

Isonicotinic acid hydrazine; antituberculotic
PRC: C

Available forms
Injection: 100 mg/ml; *Oral solution:* 50 mg/5 ml; *Tablets:* 100, 300 mg

Indications & dosages
➤ *Active tubercle bacilli*—**Adult:** 5-10 mg/kg PO or IM daily. Max 300 mg/d × 9 mo-2 yr. **Infant, child:** 10-20 mg/kg PO or IM daily. Max 300 mg/d × 18 mo-2 yr. Give with 1 other antituberculotic.
➤ *Prevent tubercle bacilli in patients exposed to TB or with nonprogressive TB*—**Adult:** 300 mg PO daily in 1 dose, continue × 6 mo. **Infant, child:** 10 mg/kg daily in 1 dose. Max 300 mg/d; continue × 6 mo.

isoproterenol (isoprenaline)
Isoproterenol, Isuprel, Vapo-Iso

isoproterenol hydrochloride
Isuprel, Norisodrine

isoproterenol sulfate
Medihaler-Iso

Adrenergic; bronchodilator, cardiac stimulant
PRC: C

Available forms
isoproterenol *Nebulizer inhaler:* 0.25, 0.5, 1%; **hydrochloride** *Aerosol inhaler:* 131 mcg/metered spray; *Injection:* 20, 200 mg/ml; *Tablets (SL):* 10, 15 mg; **sulfate** *Aerosol inhaler:* 80 mcg/metered spray

Indications & dosages
➤ *Shock*—**Adult, child:** 0.5-5 mcg/min (hydrochloride) by continuous IV infusion titrated prn.
➤ *Bronchospasm during asthma attack*—**Adult, child:** 1 inhalation (sulfate); repeat prn after 2-5 min. Max 6 inhalations daily.
➤ *Bronchospasm in COPD*—**Adult, child:** By handheld nebulizer (hydrochloride): 5-15 deep inhalations of 0.5% solution. In adult needing stronger solution, 3-7 deep inhalations of 1% solution ≤ q 3-4 hr.
➤ *Heart block, ventricular arrhythmias*—**Adult:** 0.02-0.06 mg (hydrochloride) IV; then 0.01-0.2 mg IV or 5 mcg/min IV titrated prn. Or, 0.2 mg IM; then 0.02-1 mg IM prn. **Child:** IV infusion (hydrochloride) 2.5 mcg/min or 0.1 mcg/kg/min. Titrate prn.

isosorbide dinitrate
Apo-ISDN*, Dilatrate-SR, Isonate, Isorbid, Isordil, Isordil Tembids, Isotrate, Sorbitrate

isosorbide mononitrate
Imdur, ISMO, Monoket

Nitrate; antianginal, vasodilator
PRC: C

Available forms

dinitrate *Capsules (sustained-release):* 40 mg; *Tablets:* 5, 10, 20, 30, 40 mg; *Tablets (chewable):* 5, 10 mg; *Tablets (SL):* 2.5, 5, 10 mg; *Tablets (sustained-release):* 40 mg; **mononitrate** *Tablets:* 10, 20 mg; *Tablets (extended-release):* 30, 60, 120 mg

Indications & dosages

➤ *Angina (SL, chewable tablet isosorbide dinitrate); prophylaxis for angina attacks—* **Adult:** *SL:* 2.5-10 mg; repeat q 5-10 min (max 3 doses/30 min). Prophylaxis, 2.5-10 mg q 2-3 hr. *Chewable tablets:* 5-10 mg prn, for acute attack or q 2-3 hr for prophylaxis (after initial test dose of 5 mg). *PO (dinitrate):* 5-30 mg PO tid or qid for prophylaxis; 20-40 mg PO (sustained-release) q 6-12 hr. *PO (Imdur):* 30-60 mg PO daily on arising; increase to 120 mg daily after several d prn. *PO (ISMO, Monoket):* 20 mg PO bid (give 7 hr apart).

isradipine
DynaCirc, DynaCirc CR

Calcium channel blocker; antihypertensive
PRC: C

Available forms

Capsules: 2.5, 5 mg; *Tablets (controlled-release):* 5, 10 mg

Indications & dosages

➤ *HTN—***Adult:** 2.5 mg PO bid or 5 mg PO daily (controlled-release), alone or with thiazide diuretic. If response inadequate after 1st 2-4 wk, adjust dose 5 mg daily at 2-4 wk intervals. Max 20 mg/d.

itraconazole
Sporanox

Synthetic triazole; antifungal
PRC: C

Available forms

Capsules: 100 mg; *Injection:* 10 mg/ml; *Oral solution:* 10 mg/ml

Indications & dosages

➤ *Pulmonary, extrapulmonary blastomycosis; nonmeningeal histoplasmosis—* **Adult:** 200 mg PO daily. Increase dose prn in 100-mg increments. Max 400 mg daily. Give doses > 200 mg daily in 2 divided doses. Or, 200 mg IV over 1 hr bid in 4 doses, then 200 mg IV daily. Max 14 d.†
➤ *Aspergillosis—***Adult:** 200-400 mg PO daily. Or, 200 mg IV over 1 hr bid in 4 doses, then 200 mg IV daily. Max 14 d.†
➤ *Oropharyngeal, esophageal candidiasis—***Adult:** 200 mg swished in mouth for several sec, then swallowed, daily × 1-2 wk.

ketoconazole (oral)
Nizoral

Imidazole derivative; antifungal
PRC: C

Available forms

Tablets: 200 mg

Indications & dosages

➤ *Fungal infection—***Adult:** 200 mg PO daily. Max 400 mg/d. **Child ≥ 2 yr:** 3.3-6.6 mg/kg PO daily.

---

§ Adjust in immunocompromised patients   ¶ Adjust in debilitated patients

ketoconazole (topical)
Nizoral, Nizoral A-D

Imidazole derivative; antifungal
PRC: C

Available forms
Cream, shampoo: 1%, 2%

Indications & dosages
➤ *Tinea corporis, seborrheic dermatitis, cutaneous candidiasis*—**Adult:** Cover affected and surrounding area with 2% cream daily ≥ 2 wk; for seborrheic dermatitis, apply bid × 4 wk. Shampoo 2 times/wk × 4 wk, with ≥ 3 d between shampoos prn.
➤ *Tinea infestations*—**Adult, child:** Apply daily or bid × 2 wk; tinea pedis, × 4 wk.

ketoprofen
Orudis, Orudis KT, Oruvail

NSAID; nonopioid analgesic, antipyretic, anti-inflammatory
PRC: B

Available forms
Capsules: 25, 50, 75 mg; *Capsules (extended-release):* 100, 150, 200 mg; *Tablets:* 12.5 mg

Indications & dosages
➤ *RA, OA*—**Adult:** 75 mg tid. Or, 50 mg qid or 150-200 mg (extended-release) daily. Max 300 mg/d.
➤ *Pain, dysmenorrhea*—**Adult:** 25-50 mg PO q 6-8 hr prn.
➤ *Minor aches, pain, fever*—**Adult:** 12.5 mg q 4-6 hr. Max 75 mg/24 hr.

ketorolac tromethamine (systemic)
Toradol

NSAID; analgesic
PRC: C

Available forms
Injection: 15, 30 mg/ml; *Tablets:* 10 mg

Indications & dosages
➤ *Pain*—**Adult < 65 yr:** 60 mg IM or 30 mg IV in 1 dose, or multiple doses of 30 mg IM or IV q 6 hr. Max 120 mg/d. **Elderly ≥ 65 yr:** 30 mg IM or 15 mg IV in 1 dose, or multiple doses of 15 mg IM or IV q 6 hr. Max 60 mg daily. Adjust dose in patients < 50 kg.†
➤ *Parenteral to PO treatment*—**Adult < 65 yr:** 20 mg PO in 1 dose; then 10 mg PO q 4-6 hr. Max 40 mg/d. **Elderly ≥ 65 yr or those < 50 kg:** 10 mg PO in 1 dose; then 10 mg PO q 4-6 hr. Max 40 mg/d.†

labetalol hydrochloride
Normodyne, Trandate

Alpha and beta blocker; antihypertensive
PRC: C

Available forms
Injection: 5 mg/ml; *Tablets:* 100, 200, 300 mg

Indications & dosages
➤ *HTN*—**Adult:** 100 mg PO bid with or without diuretic. May increase by 100 mg bid daily q 2-4 d prn. Maintenance 200-600 mg bid. Max 2,400 mg/d.

➤ *HTN emergencies*—**Adult:** Infuse 0.5-2 mg/min and titrate; usual cumulative dose 50-200 mg. Or, repeat IV injection 20 mg IV over 2 min. Repeat injection of 40-80 mg q 10 min to max 300 mg.

lactulose
Cephulac, Chronulac, Constulose, Duphalac, Enulose, Kristalose, Lactulax*

Disaccharide; laxative
PRC: B

Available forms
Solution: 10, 20 g/packet; *Solution (PO, PR):* 3.33 g/5 ml; *Syrup (PO):* 10 g/15 ml

Indications & dosages
➤ *Constipation*—**Adult:** 10-20 g (15-30 ml) PO daily, increase to 60 g/d prn.
➤ *Hepatic encephalopathy*—**Adult:** 20-30 g PO tid or qid until 2-3 soft BM daily. Or, 300 ml diluted with 700 ml H_2O or NSS PR and retained × 40-60 min q 4-6 hr prn.

lamivudine
Epivir, Epivir-HBV

Synthetic nucleoside analogue; antiviral
PRC: C

Available forms
Oral solution: 10 mg/ml; *Tablets:* 150, 300 mg

Indications & dosages
➤ *HIV infection*—**Adult, child ≥ 16 yr:** 300 mg PO daily or 150 mg PO bid. Give with other antiretrovirals.† **Child 3 mo-**
16 yr: 4 mg/kg PO bid. Max 150 mg bid. Give with other antiretrovirals.†
➤ *Chronic HBV infection given with other antiretrovirals*—**Adult:** 100 mg PO daily.† **Child 2-17 yr:** 3 mg/kg PO daily; max 100 mg daily.†

lamivudine and zidovudine
Combivir

Synthetic nucleoside analogue; antiviral
PRC: C

Available forms
Tablets: 150 mg lamivudine and 300 mg zidovudine

Indications & dosages
➤ *HIV infection*—**Adult, child ≥ 12 yr or > 50 kg:** 1 tablet PO bid.

lamotrigine
Lamictal

Phenyltriazine; anticonvulsant
PRC: C

Available forms
Tablets: 25, 100, 150, 200 mg; *Tablets (chewable dispersible):* 2, 5, 25 mg

Indications & dosages
➤ *Partial seizures*—**Adult, child > 12 yr:** 50 mg PO daily × 2 wk; then 100 mg/d in 2 divided doses × 2 wk. Maintenance 300-500 mg PO daily in 2 divided doses. Patients using valproic acid: 25 mg PO q other d × 2 wk; then 25 mg PO daily × 2 wk. Max 75 mg PO bid.†

---

§ Adjust in immunocompromised patients ¶Adjust in debilitated patients

lansoprazole
Prevacid, Prevacid SoluTab

Acid (proton) pump inhibitor; anti-ulcerative
PRC: B

Available forms
Capsules (delayed-release): 15, 30 mg;
Oral suspension (delayed-release): 15,
30 mg/packet; *Orally disintegrating tablets
(extended-release):* 15, 30 mg

Indications & dosages
➤ *Active duodenal ulcer*—**Adult:** 15 mg
PO daily ac × 4 wk.
➤ *Erosive esophagitis*—**Adult:** 30 mg PO
daily ac ≤ 8 wk; may give × 8 more wk
prn.
➤ *Hypersecretory conditions, including
Zollinger-Ellison syndrome*—**Adult:** 60 mg
PO daily. Increase dose prn. Give daily
doses > 120 mg in divided doses.
➤ *Reduce risk of NSAID-related ulcer in
patients with history of gastric ulcer and
need for NSAIDs*—**Adult:** 15 mg PO daily
× ≤ 12 wk.
➤ *NSAID-related ulcer in patients who
continue to take NSAIDs*—**Adult:** 30 mg
PO daily × 8 wk.
➤ *Short-term treatment of symptomatic
GERD and erosive esophagitis*—**Child 1-
11 yr ≤ 30 kg:** 15 mg PO daily for ≤ 12 wk.
Child 1-11 yr > 30 kg: 30 mg PO daily for
≤ 12 wk.

latanoprost
Xalatan

*Prostaglandin analogue; antiglaucoma
drug, ocular antihypertensive*
PRC: C

Available forms
Ophthalmic solution: 0.005% (50 mcg/ml)

Indications & dosages
➤ *First-line treatment of increased IOP in
patients with ocular HTN or open-angle
glaucoma*—**Adult:** 1 gtt in conjunctival
sac of affected eye q pm.

leflunomide
Arava

*Pyrimidine synthesis inhibitor; anti-
proliferative, anti-inflammatory*
PRC: X

Available forms
Tablets: 10, 20, 100 mg

Indications & dosages
➤ *RA*—**Adult:** 100 mg PO q 24 hr × 3 d;
then 20 mg (max daily dose) PO q 24 hr.
Reduce dose to 10 mg/d if not well tolerated.‡

leucovorin calcium
(citrovorum factor,
folinic acid)

*Formyl derivative (active reduced form of
folic acid); vitamin, antidote*
PRC: C

Available forms
Injection: 1-ml ampule (3 mg/ml with 0.9% benzyl alcohol; 10 mg/ml in 5-ml vial; 50-mg, 100-mg, and 350-mg vials for reconstitution (contain no preservatives); *Tablets:* 5, 15, 25 mg

Indications & dosages
➤ *Folic acid antagonist overdose*—**Adult, child:** IM or IV dose equivalent to wt of antagonist.
➤ *Leucovorin rescue after high methotrexate dose*—**Adult, child:** 10 mg/m² PO, IM, or IV q 6 hr until methotrexate levels < 5 × 10⁻⁸ M.
➤ *Megaloblastic anemia from congenital enzyme deficiency*—**Adult, child:** 3-6 mg IM daily.
➤ *Folate-deficient megaloblastic anemia*—**Adult, child:** ≤ 1 mg IM daily.

levetiracetam
Keppra

Antiepileptic; anticonvulsant
PRC: C

Available forms
Tablets: 250, 500, 750 mg

Indications & dosages
➤ *Partial onset seizures*—**Adult:** 500 mg PO bid. Increase by 500 mg PO bid q 2 wk prn; max 1,500 mg PO bid.†

levodopa
Dopar, Larodopa

Dopamine precursor; antiparkinsonian
PRC: C

Available forms
Capsules: 100, 250, 500 mg; *Tablets:* 100, 250, 500 mg

Indications & dosages
Parkinsonism—**Adult:** 0.5-1 g PO daily divided bid, tid, or qid with food; increase by 100-750 mg q 3-7 d; usual dose 3-6 g daily divided into 3 doses. Max 8 g/d except in rare patients.

levodopa-carbidopa
Sinemet, Sinemet CR

Decarboxylase inhibitor, dopamine precursor; antiparkinsonian
PRC: C

Available forms
Tablets: carbidopa 10 mg and levodopa 100 mg (Sinemet 10-100), carbidopa 25 mg and levodopa 100 mg (Sinemet 25-100), carbidopa 25 mg and levodopa 250 mg (Sinemet 25-250); *Tablets (extended-release):* carbidopa 50 mg and levodopa 200 mg, carbidopa 25 mg and levodopa 100 mg (Sinemet CR)

Indications & dosages
➤ *Parkinson's disease, symptomatic parkinsonism*—**Adult:** 1 tablet 25 mg carbidopa and 100 mg levodopa PO tid; increase by 1 tablet daily or q other d prn,

to max 8 tablets daily (25 mg carbidopa and 250 mg levodopa or 10 mg carbidopa and 100 mg levodopa tablet substituted prn, for max response). *Extended-release:* Dose calculated on current levodopa intake. Initially, extended-release dose should amount to 10% more levodopa per d; increase prn to 30% more per d in divided doses q 4-8 hr.

levofloxacin
Levaquin

Fluoroquinolone; antibiotic
PRC: C

Available forms
Single-use vials: 500 mg; *Infusion (premixed in D_5W):* 250 mg/50 ml, 500 mg/100 ml, 750 mg/150 ml; *Tablets:* 250, 500, 750 mg

Indications & dosages
➤ *Maxillary sinusitis*—**Adult:** 500 mg PO or IV daily × 10-14 d.†
➤ *Exacerbation of chronic bronchitis*—**Adult:** 500 mg PO or IV daily × 7 d.†
➤ *Complicated skin infection*—**Adult:** 750 mg PO or IV q 24 hr × 7-14 d.†
➤ *Uncomplicated UTI*—**Adult:** 250 mg PO daily × 3 d.
➤ *Uncomplicated skin infection*—**Adult:** 500 mg PO or IV daily × 7-10 d.†
➤ *Complicated UTI, acute pyelonephritis*—**Adult:** 250 mg PO or IV q 24 h × 10 d.†
➤ *Community-acquired pneumonia caused by PCN-resistant* Streptococcus pneumoniae—**Adult:** 500 mg PO or IV infusion over 60 min once daily × 7-14 d.†

➤ *Nosocomial pneumonia*—**Adult:** 750 mg PO or IV daily × 7-14 d.†
➤ *Chronic bacterial prostatitis*—**Adult:** 500 mg PO or IV daily × 28 d.†

levothyroxine sodium (T_4 or L-thyroxine sodium)
Eltroxin*, Levo-T, Levothroid, Levoxine, Levoxyl, Novothyrox, Synthroid, Thyro-Tabs, Unithroid

Thyroid hormone; thyroid hormone replacement
PRC: A

Available forms
Injection: 200, 500 mcg/vial; *Tablets:* 25, 50, 75, 88, 100, 112, 125, 137, 150, 175, 200, 300 mcg

Indications & dosages
➤ *Myxedema coma*—**Adult:** 200-500 mcg IV; if no response in 24 hr, 100-300 mcg IV. Maintenance 50-200 mcg IV daily.
➤ *Thyroid hormone replacement*—**Adult:** 50 mcg PO daily; increase by 25-50 mcg PO daily q 2-4 wk. May give IV or IM. **Adult > 65 yr:** 12.5-50 mcg PO daily. Increase by 12.5-25 mcg q 2-8 wk prn. **Child > 12 yr:** > 150 mcg or 2-3 mcg/kg/d. **Child 6-12 yr:** 100-150 mcg or 4-5 mcg/kg/d. **Child 1-5 yr:** 75-100 mcg or 5-6 mcg/kg/d. **Child 6-12 mo:** 50-75 mcg or 6-8 mcg/kg/d. **Child < 6 mo:** 25-50 mcg or 8-10 mcg/kg/d.

---

lidocaine hydrochloride (lignocaine hydrochloride)
LidoPen Auto-Injector, Xylocaine

Amide derivative; ventricular antiarrhythmic, local anesthetic
PRC: B

Available forms
Infusion (premixed): 0.2% (2 mg/ml), 0.4% (4 mg/ml), 0.8% (8 mg/ml); *Injection (IM):* 300 mg/3 ml automatic injection device; *Injection (direct IV):* 1% (10 mg/ml), 2% (20 mg/ml); *Injection (IV admixtures):* 4% (40 mg/ml), 10% (100 mg/ml), 20% (200 mg/ml)

Indications & dosages
➤ *Ventricular arrhythmias*—**Adult:** 50-100 mg (1-1.5 mg/kg) IV bolus at 25-50 mg/min. Repeat bolus dose q 5-10 min prn or as tolerated. Max 300-mg total bolus over 1 hr. At same time, begin infusion of 20-50 mcg/kg/min (1-4 mg/min). **Elderly:** Reduce dose and rate of infusion by 50%. **Child:** 0.5-1 mg/kg IV bolus; then infusion of 10-50 mcg/kg/min. Adjust dose in patients < 50 kg or with HF.†,‡

linezolid
Zyvox

Oxazolidinone; antibiotic
PRC: C

Available forms
Injection: 2 mg/ml; *Powder for oral suspension:* 100 mg/5 ml (reconstituted); *Tablets:* 400, 600 mg

Indications & dosages
➤ *Vancomycin-resistant* Enterococcus faecium *infections, including those with concurrent bacteremia*—**Adult, child ≥ 12 yr:** 600 mg IV or PO q 12 hr × 14-28 d. **Neonate ≥ 7 d, infant, child < 12 yr:** 10 mg/kg IV or PO q 8 hr × 14-28 d. **Neonate < 7 d:** 10 mg/kg IV or PO q 12 hr. Increase to 10 mg/kg q 8 hr when patient is 7 d old or has subclinical response.
➤ *Nosocomial pneumonia, complicated skin and skin-structure infections, community-acquired pneumonia including those with concurrent bacteremia*—**Adult, child ≥ 12 yr:** 600 mg IV or PO q 12 hr × 10-14 d. **Neonate ≥ 7 d, infant, child < 12 yr:** 10 mg/kg IV or PO q 8 hr × 10-14 d. **Neonate < 7 d:** 10 mg/kg IV or PO q 12 hr. Increase to 10 mg/kg q 8 hr when patient is 7 d old or has subclinical response.
➤ *Uncomplicated skin and skin-structure infections from* Staphylococcus aureus *(MSSA only) or* Streptococcus pyogenes—**Adult:** 400 mg PO q 12 hr × 10-14 d. **Child 12-18 yr:** 600 mg PO q 12 hr × 10-14 d. **Child 5-11 yr:** 10 mg/kg PO q 12 hr × 10-14 d. **Neonate ≥ 7 d, infant, child < 5 yr:** 10 mg/kg PO q 8 hr × 10-14 d. **Neonate < 7 d:** 10 mg/kg IV or PO q 12 hr. Increase to 10 mg/kg q 8 hr when patient is 7 d old or has subclinical response.

lisinopril
Prinivil, Zestril

ACE inhibitor; antihypertensive
PRC: C (D, 2nd and 3rd trimesters)

Available forms
Tablets: 2.5, 5, 10, 20, 40 mg

---

§ Adjust in immunocompromised patients   ¶ Adjust in debilitated patients

Indications & dosages
➤ *HTN*—**Adult:** 5-10 mg PO daily. Usually 20-40 mg daily. Adjust dose in patients taking diuretics.
➤ *HF (with diuretics and cardiac glycosides)*—**Adult:** 5 mg PO daily. Usually 5-20 mg/d.
➤ *Acute MI*—**Adult:** 5 mg PO; then 5 mg in 24 hr, 10 mg in 48 hr; then 10 mg/d × 6 wk. In patients with systolic BP ≤ 120 when treatment begins or during first 3 d after MI, reduce to 2.5 mg PO. If systolic BP ≤ 100, reduce maintenance dose from 5 to 2.5 mg/d.

lithium carbonate
Carbolith*, Eskalith CR, Lithobid, Lithonate, Lithotabs

lithium citrate
Cibalith-S

Alkali metal; antimanic, antipsychotic
PRC: D

Available forms
carbonate *Capsules:* 150, 300, 600 mg; *Tablets:* 300 mg (300 mg = 8.12 mEq lithium); *Tablets (controlled-release):* 300, 450 mg; **citrate** *Syrup (sugarless):* 8 mEq (lithium)/5 ml. *Note:* 5 ml lithium citrate contains 8 mEq lithium = 300 mg lithium carbonate

Indications & dosages
➤ *Mania*—**Adult:** 300-600 mg PO up to qid, or 900 mg (Eskalith CR tablet) PO q 12 hr; increase based on blood levels prn.

loperamide
Imodium A-D, Kaopectate II Caplets

Piperidine derivative; antidiarrheal
PRC: B

Available forms
Capsules, caplets: 2 mg; *Oral liq:* 1 mg/5 ml

Indications & dosages
➤ *Diarrhea*—**Adult, child ≥ 12 yr:** 4 mg PO; then 2 mg after each unformed BM. Max 16 mg daily. **Child 9-11 yr:** 2 mg PO tid, d 1. **Child 6-8 yr:** 2 mg PO bid, d 1. **Child 2-5 yr:** 1 mg PO tid, d 1. Maintenance ⅓-½ initial dose for child < 11 yr.

lopinavir and ritonavir
Kaletra

Protease inhibitor; antiviral
PRC: C

Available forms
Capsules: lopinavir 133.3 mg and ritonavir 33.3 mg; *Solution:* lopinavir 400 mg and ritonavir 100 mg/5 ml (80 mg/20 mg per ml)

Indications & dosages
➤ *HIV infection (used with other antiretrovirals)*—**Adult, child > 12 yr:** 400 mg lopinavir and 100 mg ritonavir (3 capsules or 5 ml) PO bid with food. If susceptibility to lopinavir is suspected, consider dose of 533 mg and 133 mg (4 capsules or 6.5 ml) PO bid with food. **Child 6 mo-12 yr and 15-40 kg:** 10 mg/kg (lopinavir content) PO bid with food; max 400/

100 mg in child > 40 kg. If reduced susceptibility to lopinavir is suspected, consider dose of 11 mg/kg (lopinavir content) PO bid. Treatment-experienced child > 50 kg can receive adult dose. **Child 6 mo-12 yr and 7 to < 15 kg:** 12 mg/kg (lopinavir content) PO bid with food. If reduced susceptibility to lopinavir is suspected, consider dose of 13 mg/kg (lopinavir content) PO bid with food.

loracarbef
Lorabid

Synthetic beta-lactam antibiotic (carbacephem class); antibiotic
PRC: B

Available forms
Powder for oral suspension: 100, 200 mg/5 ml in 50-, 100-ml bottles; *Pulvules:* 200, 400 mg

Indications & dosages
➤ *Secondary infection of acute bronchitis*—**Adult:** 200-400 mg PO q 12 hr × 7 d.†
➤ *Exacerbation of chronic bronchitis*—**Adult:** 400 mg PO q 12 hr × 7 d.†
➤ *Pneumonia*—**Adult:** 400 mg PO q 12 hr × 14 d.†
➤ *Pharyngitis, sinusitis, tonsillitis*—**Adult:** 200 mg PO q 12 hr × 10 d. **Child:** 15 mg/kg PO daily in divided doses q 12 hr × 10 d.†
➤ *OM*—**Child:** 15 mg/kg (oral suspension) PO q 12 hr × 10 d.†

loratadine
Alavert, Claritin, Tavist ND Allergy

Tricyclic antihistamine; antihistaminic
PRC: B

Available forms
Syrup: 1 mg/ml; *Tablets:* 10 mg; *Tablets (rapidly disintegrating):* 10 mg

Indications & dosages
➤ *Seasonal allergic rhinitis, urticaria*—**Adult, child ≥ 6 yr:** 10 mg PO daily.†,‡ **Child 2-5 yr:** 5 mg PO daily.

lorazepam
Alzapam, Apo-Lorazepam*, Ativan, Lorazepam Intensol, Novo-Lorazem*, Nu-Loraz*

Benzodiazepine; anxiolytic, sedative-hypnotic
PRC: D; CSS: IV

Available forms
Injection: 2, 4 mg/ml; *Oral solution (concentrate):* 2 mg/ml; *Tablets:* 0.5, 1, 2 mg; *Tablets (SL):* 0.5*, 1*, 2 mg

Indications & dosages
➤ *Anxiety, agitation, irritability*—**Adult:** 2-6 mg PO daily in divided doses. Max 10 mg daily. Or, 0.05 mg/kg up to 4 mg IM daily in divided doses, or 0.044-0.05 mg/kg up to 4 mg IV daily in divided doses.
➤ *Insomnia*—**Adult:** 2-4 mg PO hs.
➤ *Preop sedation*—**Adult:** 0.05 mg/kg IM 2 hr preop. Max 4 mg. Or, 0.044 mg/kg,

---

max 2 mg IV, 15-20 min preop. **Adult < 50 yr:** May give 0.05 mg/kg; max 4 mg.

losartan potassium
Cozaar

Angiotensin II receptor antagonist; antihypertensive
PRC: C (D, 2nd and 3rd trimesters)

Available forms
Tablets: 25, 50, 100 mg

Indications & dosages
➤ *HTN*—**Adult:** 25-50 mg PO daily. Max 100 mg daily in 1 dose or divided bid. Adjust dose in patients with intravascular volume depletion.‡
➤ *Nephropathy in type 2 DM*—**Adult:** 50 mg PO daily. Increase to 100 mg daily based on BP response.
➤ *Reduce risk of stroke in patients with HTN and left ventricular hypertrophy*—**Adult:** 50 mg PO daily; adjust based on BP and add hydrochlorothiazide 12.5 mg PO daily.

lovastatin (mevinolin)
Altocor, Mevacor

HMG-CoA reductase inhibitor; antilipemic
PRC: X

Available forms
Tablets: 10, 20, 40 mg; *Tablets (extended-release):* 10, 20, 40, 60 mg

Indications & dosages
➤ *Primary prevention and treatment of CAD; hyperlipidemia*—**Adult:** 20 mg PO daily with pm meal. Dose range 10-80 mg daily or divided bid. Or, 20-60 mg (extended-release) PO hs. Starting dose of 10 mg can be used for patients requiring smaller reductions. For patients also taking cyclosporine, 10 mg PO daily. Max 20 mg daily. Don't exceed 20 mg daily in patients also taking fibrates or niacin.†
➤ *Heterozygous familial hypercholesterolemia*—**Child 10-17 yr (girls should be ≥ 1 yr postmenarche):** 10-40 mg/d PO with pm meal. Patients requiring ≥ 20% reduction in LDL–cholesterol complex, start with 20 mg/d.

magnesium chloride
Slow-Mag

magnesium sulfate

Mineral, electrolyte; nutritional supplement
PRC: NR

Available forms
chloride *Injection:* 20% in 50-ml vial; *Tablets (delayed-release):* 64 mg; **sulfate** *Injection solution:* 10, 12.5, 50% in 2-, 5-, 10-, 20-, 30-, 50-ml ampules, vials, prefilled syringes

Indications & dosages
➤ *Hypomagnesemia*—**Adult:** 1 g (50% solution) IM q 6 hr × 4 doses, depending on serum magnesium level. Or, 3 g PO q 6 hr × 4 doses.
➤ *Severe symptomatic hypomagnesemia (serum magnesium ≤ 0.8 mEq/L)*—**Adult:** 5 g IV in 1 L solution over 3 hr, then reevaluate.

➤ *Magnesium supplementation*—**Adult:** 2 tablets PO daily, or as much as 2 mEq/ kg IM within 4 hr prn. As part of total parenteral nutrition, 5-8 mEq daily.

magnesium citrate (citrate of magnesia)
Citroma, Citro-Mag*, Citro-Nesia, Evac-Q-Mag

magnesium hydroxide (milk of magnesia)
Milk of Magnesia, Phillips' Chewable, Phillips' Milk of Magnesia

magnesium sulfate (epsom salts)

Magnesium salt; antacid, antiulcerative, laxative
PRC: NR

Available forms
citrate *Oral solution:* About 1.75 g magnesium/30 ml; **hydroxide** *Oral suspension:* 400, 800 mg/5 ml; *Tablets, chewable:* 311 mg; **sulfate** *Granules:* About 40 mEq magnesium/5 g

Indications & dosages
➤ *Constipation, bowel evacuation*—**Adult, child ≥ 12 yr:** 11-25 g citrate PO daily; 2.4-4.8 g (30-60 ml) hydroxide PO daily; 10-30 g sulfate PO daily. **Child 6-12 yr:** 5.5-12.5 g citrate PO daily; 1.2-2.4 g (15-30 ml) hydroxide PO daily; 5-10 g sulfate PO daily. **Child 2-6 yr:** 2.7-6.25 g citrate PO daily; 0.4-1.2 g (5-15 ml) hydroxide PO daily; 2.5-5 g sulfate PO daily. *Note:* All doses may be single or divided.

➤ *Antacid*—**Adult, child > 12 yr:** 5-15 ml hydroxide PO qid, or 622-1244 mg qid.

magnesium oxide
Mag-Ox 400, Maox 420, Uro-Mag

Magnesium salt; antacid, laxative
PRC: NR

Available forms
Capsules: 140 mg; *Tablets:* 400, 420, 500 mg

Indications & dosages
➤ *Antacid*—**Adult:** 140 mg PO with H_2O or milk pc and hs.
➤ *Laxative*—**Adult:** 4 g PO with H_2O or milk, usually hs.
➤ *Hypomagnesemia*—**Adult:** 400-840 mg PO daily.

magnesium sulfate

Mineral, electrolyte; anticonvulsant
PRC: A

Available forms
Injection: 4, 8, 10, 12.5, 25, 50%; *Injection solution:* 1, 2% in D_5W

Indications & dosages
➤ *Seizures in preeclampsia or eclampsia*—**Adult:** 4 g IV in 250 ml D_5W and 4-5 g deep IM each buttock; then 4 g deep IM alternate buttock q 4 hr prn. Or, 4 g IV initially; then 1-2 g/hr IV infusion. Max 40 g/d.
➤ *Hypomagnesemia, seizures*—**Adult:** 1-2 g (as 10% solution) IV over 15 min;

then 1 g IM q 4-6 hr, per response and drug levels.

➤ *Seizures, hypomagnesemia with acute nephritis in child*—**Child:** 0.2 ml/kg 50% solution IM q 4-6 hr prn, or 100-200 mg/kg 1-3% solution IV slowly.

➤ *PAT*—**Adult:** 3-4 g IV over 30 sec.

➤ *Ventricular arrhythmias*—**Adult:** 1-6 g IV over several min, then 3-20 mg/min IV × 5-48 hr.

mannitol
Osmitrol

Osmotic diuretic; diuretic
PRC: B

Available forms
Injection: 5, 10, 15, 20, 25%

Indications & dosages
➤ *Test dose for oliguria or inadequate renal function*—**Adult, child > 12 yr:** 200 mg/kg or 12.5 g as 15% or 20% IV solution over 3-5 min. Response is adequate if 30-50 ml/hr urine is produced in 2-3 hr; if inadequate, give 2nd test dose. Stop if there is no response.

➤ *Oliguria*—**Adult, child > 12 yr:** 100 g IV usually as 15% or 20% solution over 1½ to several hr.

meclizine hydrochloride
Antivert, Bonamine*, Bonine, Dramamine Less Drowsy Formula, Meni-D, Vergon

Piperazine-derivative antihistamine; antiemetic, antivertigo drug
PRC: B

Available forms
Capsules: 25, 30 mg; *Tablets:* 12.5, 25, 50 mg; *Tablets (chewable):* 25 mg

Indications & dosages
➤ *Vertigo*—**Adult:** 25-100 mg PO daily in divided doses.

➤ *Motion sickness*—**Adult:** 25-50 mg PO 1 hr before travel, then daily during trip.

medroxyprogesterone acetate
Amen, Curretab, Cycrin, Depo-Provera, Provera

Progestin; antineoplastic, hormonal contraceptive
PRC: X

Available forms
Injection (suspension): 150, 400 mg/ml; *Tablets:* 2.5, 5, 10 mg

Indications & dosages
➤ *Abnormal uterine bleeding*—**Adult:** 5-10 mg PO daily × 5-10 d starting on d 16 of menstrual cycle. If patient using estrogen, 10 mg PO daily × 10 d starting on d 16 of cycle.

➤ *Secondary amenorrhea*—**Adult:** 5-10 mg PO daily × 5-10 d.

➤ *Endometrial or renal CA*—**Adult:** 400-1,000 mg IM wkly.

➤ *Contraception*—**Adult:** 150 mg IM q 3 mo; give 1st injection during 1st 5 d of menstrual cycle.

medroxyprogesterone acetate and estradiol cypionate
Lunelle

Estrogen and progestin; combined hormonal contraceptive
PRC: X

Available forms
Injection: 25 mg medroxyprogesterone acetate and 5 mg estradiol cypionate per 0.5 ml

Indications & dosages
➤ *Contraception*—**Women > 16 yr who have had menarche:** 0.5 ml IM. Give 1st dose within 1st 5 d of onset of normal menstrual period, within 5 d of a complete 1st trimester abortion, or ≥ 4 wk postpartum if not breast-feeding (≥ 6 wk postpartum if breast-feeding). Give 2nd and subsequent doses q mo (28-30 d, ≤ 33 d) after previous dose.

megestrol acetate
Megace

Progestin; antineoplastic
PRC: D

Available forms
Oral suspension: 40 mg/ml; *Tablets:* 20, 40 mg

Indications & dosages
➤ *Breast CA*—**Adult:** 40 mg PO qid.
➤ *Endometrial CA*—**Adult:** 40-320 mg PO daily in divided doses.

➤ *Significant wt loss*—**Adult:** 800 mg PO (oral suspension) daily.

meloxicam
Mobic

Enolic acid NSAID; anti-inflammatory, analgesic
PRC: C

Available forms
Tablets: 7.5 mg

Indications & dosages
➤ *OA*—**Adult:** 7.5 mg PO daily. Increase prn. Max 15 mg/d.

meperidine hydrochloride (pethidine hydrochloride)
Demerol

Opioid; analgesic, adjunct to anesthesia
PRC: C; CSS II

Available forms
Injection: 10, 25, 50, 75, 100 mg/ml; *Syrup:* 50 mg/5 ml; *Tablets:* 50, 100 mg

Indications & dosages
➤ *Pain*—**Adult:** 50-150 mg PO, IM, IV, or SC q 3-4 hr. **Child:** 1.1-1.8 mg/kg PO, IM, IV, or SC q 3-4 hr, or 175 mg/m² daily in 6 divided doses. Max single dose ≤ 100 mg.†,‡,¶
➤ *Preop*—**Adult:** 50-100 mg IM, IV, or SC 30-90 min preop. **Child:** 1-2.2 mg/kg IM, IV, or SC up to adult dose 30-90 min preop.

§ Adjust in immunocompromised patients ¶ Adjust in debilitated patients

metaproterenol sulfate
Alupent

Adrenergic; bronchodilator
PRC: C

Available forms
Aerosol inhaler: 0.65 mg/metered spray;
Nebulizer inhaler: 0.4, 0.6, 5% solution;
Syrup: 10 mg/5 ml; *Tablets:* 10, 20 mg

Indications & dosages
➤ *Asthma*—**Adult, child ≥ 12 yr:** 2-3 inhalations q 3-4 hr. Max 12 inhalations daily.
➤ *Asthma and reversible bronchospasm*—**Adult, child > 9 yr or > 27 kg:** 20 mg PO q 6-8 hr. **Child 6-9 yr or < 27 kg:** 10 mg PO q 6-8 hr. **Child < 6 yr:** 1.3-2.6 mg/kg/d PO in divided doses. Or, via IPPB or nebulizer: **Adult, child ≥ 12 yr:** 0.2-0.3 ml 5% solution diluted in 2.5 ml ½ NSS or NSS, or 2.5 ml 0.4% or 0.6% solution q 4 hr prn. **Child 6-12 yr:** 0.1-0.2 ml 5% solution diluted in NSS to 3 ml q 4 hr prn.

metformin hydrochloride
Glucophage, Glucophage XR

Biguanide; antidiabetic
PRC: B

Available forms
Tablets: 500, 850, 1,000 mg; *Tablets (extended-release):* 500, 750 mg

Indications & dosages
➤ *Type 2 DM*—**Adult:** 500 mg PO bid with am, pm meals; or 850 mg PO daily with am meal. With 500 mg, increase dose 500 mg/wk to max 2,500 mg PO daily in divided doses prn. With 850 mg, increase dose 850 mg q other wk to max 2,550 mg PO daily in divided doses prn. Use lower dose in elderly. If using extended-release form, start with 500 mg PO daily with pm meal. May increase in wkly increments of 500 mg; max 2,000 mg/d. **Child 10-16 yr:** 500 mg PO (regular-release only) bid; increase in 500-mg increments wkly to max 2,000 mg/d in divided doses.¶

methadone hydrochloride
Dolophine, Methadose

Opioid; analgesic, opioid detoxification adjunct
PRC: C; CSS: II

Available forms
Injection: 10 mg/ml; *Dispersible tablets (methadone maintenance treatment):* 40 mg; *Oral solution:* 5, 10 mg/5 ml, 10 mg/10 ml, 10 mg/1 ml (concentrate); *Tablets:* 5, 10 mg

Indications & dosages
➤ *Pain*—**Adult:** 2.5-10 mg PO, IM, or SC q 3-4 hr prn.
➤ *Opioid withdrawal syndrome*—**Adult:** 15-40 mg PO daily. Maintenance 20-120 mg PO daily. Doses > 120 mg/d need state, federal approval.

methotrexate (amethopterin, MTX)

methotrexate sodium
Folex PFS, Mexate-AQ, Rheumatrex

Antimetabolite (cell cycle-phase specific, S phase); antineoplastic, immunosuppressant
PRC: X

Available forms
Injection: 20-, 25-, 50-, 100-, 250-mg vials, lyophilized powder, preservative free; 25-mg/ml vials, preservative-free solution; 2.5-, 25-mg/ml vials, lyophilized powder, preserved; *Tablets (scored):* 2.5 mg

Indications & dosages
➤ *Trophoblastic tumors*—**Adult:** 15-30 mg PO or IM daily × 5 d. Repeat after ≥ 1 wk, based on response or toxicity.†
➤ *ALL*—**Adult, child:** 3.3 mg/m²/d PO, IM, or IV daily × 4-6 wk or until remission; then 20-30 mg/m² PO or IM wkly in 2 divided doses or 2.5 mg/kg IV q 14 d.†
➤ *Meningeal leukemia*—**Adult, child:** ≤ 12 mg/m² (max 15 mg) intrathecally q 2-5 d until CSF is normal; then 1 more dose.†
➤ *RA*—**Adult:** Initially, 7.5 mg/wk PO as single dose or divided into 2.5 mg PO q 12 hr × 3 doses wkly. Increase gradually to optimum response. Don't exceed 20 mg/wk. Reduce to lowest effective dose.†

methyldopa
Aldomet, Apo-Methyldopa*, Dopamet*, Novo-Medopa*

methyldopate hydrochloride
Aldomet

Centrally acting antiadrenergic; antihypertensive
PRC: B

Available forms
methyldopa *Oral suspension:* 250 mg/ 5 ml; *Tablets:* 125, 250, 500 mg; **hydrochloride** *Injection:* 250 mg/5 ml

Indications & dosages
➤ *HTN, HTN crisis*—**Adult:** 250 mg PO bid or tid in 1st 48 hr. Increase prn q 2 d. Maintenance 500 mg-3 g daily in 2-4 divided doses; max 3 g/d. Or, 250-500 mg diluted in D₅W IV over 30-60 min q 6 hr; max dose 1 g q 6 hr. **Child:** 10 mg/kg PO daily in 2-4 divided doses; or 20-40 mg/ kg IV daily in 4 divided doses. Increase dose daily prn. Max 65 mg/kg or 3 g daily.

methylphenidate hydrochloride
Concerta, Metadate CD, Metadate ER, Methylin, Methylin ER, PMS-Methylphenidate*, Ritalin, Ritalin LA, Ritalin-SR

Piperidine CNS stimulant; CNS stimulant (analeptic)
PRC: NR (C, Concerta, Metadate CD, Ritalin LA); CSS: II

---

§ Adjust in immunocompromised patients   ¶ Adjust in debilitated patients

Available forms

Capsules: 20 mg; *Capsules (extended-release):* 20, 30, 40 mg; *Oral solution:* 5, 10 mg/5 ml; *Tablets:* 5, 10, 20 mg; *Tablets (extended-release):* 10, 18, 20, 27, 36, 54 mg; *Tablets (sustained-release):* 20 mg

Indications & dosages

➤ *ADHD (Metadate ER, Methylin, Methylin ER, Ritalin, Ritalin-SR)*—**Child ≥ 6 yr:** 5-10 mg PO daily before breakfast and lunch; increase in 5- to 10-mg increments wkly prn; max 2 mg/kg or 60 mg/d.
➤ *ADHD (Metadate CD)*—**Child ≥ 6 yr:** 20 mg PO daily before breakfast; increase in 20-mg increments wkly to max of 60 mg/d.
➤ *ADHD (Ritalin LA)*—**Child ≥ 6 yr:** 20 mg PO daily. Adjust dosage in wkly 10-mg increments to max of 60 mg daily. If previous daily dose is 10 mg bid or 20 mg sustained-release, give 20 mg PO daily. If previous daily dose is 15 mg bid, give 30 mg PO daily. If previous daily dose is 20 mg bid or 40 mg sustained-release, give 40 mg PO daily. If previous daily dose is 30 mg bid or 60 mg sustained-release, give 60 mg PO daily.
➤ *ADHD (Concerta)*—**Child ≥ 6 yr not taking drug or taking stimulants:** Initially, 18 mg PO daily in am. Adjust wkly by 18-mg increments to max of 54 mg PO daily in am. **Child ≥ 6 yr taking this drug:** If previous daily dose is 10-15 mg or 20 mg sustained-release, give 18 mg PO q am. If previous daily dose is 20-30 mg or 40 mg sustained-release, give 36 mg PO q am. If previous daily dose 30-45 mg or 60 mg sustained-release, give 54 mg

PO q am. Adjust in 18-mg increments q wk prn. Max 54 mg/d.
➤ *Narcolepsy (Metadate ER, Methylin, Methylin ER, Ritalin, Ritalin-SR)*—**Adult:** 10 mg PO bid or tid 30-45 min ac. Some patients may require 40-60 mg/d.
Note: Ritalin-SR, Metadate ER, and Methylin ER tablets may be used in place of methylphenidate tablets by calculating the dose of methylphenidate in intervals of 8 hr.

methylprednisolone
Medrol

methylprednisolone acetate
depMedalone 40, depMedalone 80, Depo-Medrol, Depopred-40, Depopred-80

methylprednisolone sodium succinate
A-MethaPred, Solu-Medrol

Glucocorticoid; anti-inflammatory, immunosuppressant
PRC: C

Available forms

methylprednisolone *Tablets:* 2, 4, 8, 16, 24, 32 mg; **acetate** *Injection (suspension):* 20, 40, 80 mg/ml; **sodium succinate** *Injection:* 40-, 125-, 500-, 1,000-, 2,000-mg vials

Indications & dosages

➤ *MS*—**Adult:** 200 mg PO daily × 1 wk; then 80 mg q other d × 1 mo.

➤ *Inflammation, immunosuppression*—**Adult:** 2-60 mg PO daily in 4 divided doses; or 10-80 mg acetate IM daily, or 10-250 mg succinate IM or IV up to q 4 hr. Or, 4-40 mg acetate into small joints or 20-80 mg acetate into large joints. **Child:** 0.03-0.2 mg/kg succinate or 1-6.25 mg/m² IM daily or bid.

➤ *Shock*—**Adult:** 100-250 mg succinate IV at 2-6 hr intervals; or 30 mg/kg IV, repeated q 4-6 hr prn. Continue treatment × 2-3 d or until patient is stable.

metoclopramide hydrochloride
Apo-Metoclop*, Clopra, Maxolon, Metoclopramide Intensol, Octamide, Reclomide, Reglan

Para-aminobenzoic acid derivative; antiemetic, GI stimulant
PRC: B

Available forms
Injection: 5 mg/ml; *Oral solution:* 5 mg/5 ml, 10 mg/ml (concentrate); *Tablets:* 5, 10 mg

Indications & dosages
➤ *Nausea, vomiting with chemo*—**Adult:** 1-2 mg/kg IV 30 min before chemo; repeat q 2 hr × 2 doses, then q 3 hr × 3 doses.

➤ *Postop nausea, vomiting*—**Adult:** 10-20 mg IM near end of procedure; then q 4-6 hr prn.

➤ *Small bowel intubation, aid in radiologic exams*—**Adult, child > 14 yr:** 10 mg IV × 1 dose over 1-2 min. **Child 6-14 yr:** 2.5-5 mg IV. **Child < 6 yr:** 0.1 mg/kg IV.

➤ *GERD*—**Adult:** 10-15 mg PO qid prn, 30 min ac and hs.

metolazone
Mykrox, Zaroxolyn

Quinazoline derivative (thiazide-like) diuretic; diuretic, antihypertensive
PRC: B

Available forms
Tablets (extended-release): 2.5, 5, 10 mg (Zaroxolyn); *Tablets (prompt-release):* 0.5 mg (Mykrox)

Indications & dosages
➤ *Edema*—**Adult:** 5-20 mg (extended-release) PO daily.

➤ *HTN*—**Adult:** 2.5-5 mg (extended-release) PO daily. Maintenance based on BP. Or, 0.5 mg (prompt-release) PO daily in am; increase to 1 mg PO daily.

metoprolol succinate
Toprol-XL

metoprolol tartrate
Apo-Metoprolol*, Lopressor

Beta blocker; antihypertensive, adjunctive treatment for acute MI
PRC: C

Available forms
succinate *Tablets (extended-release):* 25, 50, 100, 200 mg; **tartrate** *Injection:* 1 mg/ml in 5-ml ampule; *Tablets:* 50, 100 mg

---

§ Adjust in immunocompromised patients   ¶ Adjust in debilitated patients

Indications & dosages
➤ *HTN*—**Adult:** 100 mg PO in 1 dose or divided doses; maintenance 100-450 mg/d in 2-3 divided doses. Or, 50-100 mg extended-release tablet daily; max 400 mg/d.
➤ *Acute MI*—**Adult:** 5-mg (tartrate) IV bolus q 2 min × 3 doses. Then, 15 min after last dose, 25-50 mg PO q 6 hr × 48 hr. Maintenance 100 mg PO bid.
➤ *Angina*—**Adult:** 100 mg PO daily in 2 divided doses or 100 mg extended-release tablet daily. Maintenance 100-400 mg/d.
➤ *Stable, symptomatic HF from ischemia, HTN, or cardiomyopathy*—**Adult:** 25 mg extended-release tablet PO daily × 2 wk. Double dose q 2 wk as tolerated to max of 200 mg daily. In patient with more severe HF, start with 12.5 mg PO daily × 2 wk.

metronidazole (systemic)
Apo-Metronidazole*, Flagyl, Protostat, Trikacide*

metronidazole hydrochloride
Flagyl IV RTU, Metro IV, Novonidazol*

Nitroimidazole; antibacterial, antiprotozoal, amebicide
PRC: B

Available forms
Capsules: 375 mg; *Injection:* 5 mg/ml; *Powder for injection:* 500-mg single-dose vial; *Tablets:* 250, 500 mg; *Tablets (extended-release):* 750 mg

Indications & dosages
➤ *Intestinal amebiasis*—**Adult:** 750 mg PO tid × 5-10 d. **Child:** 30-50 mg/kg/d (in 3 doses) × 10 d.
➤ *Trichomoniasis*—**Adult:** 250 mg PO tid × 7 d or 2 g PO in 1 dose; repeat after 4-6 wk. **Child:** 5 mg/kg dose PO tid × 7 d.
➤ *Refractory trichomoniasis*—**Adult:** 250 or 500 mg PO bid × 10 or 7 d, respectively.
➤ *Bacterial infection from anaerobic microorganisms*—**Adult:** Loading 15 mg/kg IV over 1 hr. Maintenance 7.5 mg/kg IV or PO q 6 hr. First maintenance dose 6 hr after loading dose. Max 4 g/d.
➤ *Contaminated colorectal surgery*—**Adult:** 15 mg/kg IV over 30-60 min 1 hr preop; then 7.5 mg/kg IV over 30-60 min at 6 and 12 hr after 1st dose.

mexiletine hydrochloride
Mexitil

Lidocaine analogue, sodium channel antagonist; ventricular antiarrhythmic
PRC: C

Available forms
Capsules: 100*, 150, 200, 250 mg

Indications & dosages
➤ *Ventricular arrhythmias*—**Adult:** 200 mg PO q 8 hr. May increase to 50-100 mg q 8 hr. Or, loading dose 400 mg with maintenance dose 200 mg q 8 hr. Max 1,200 mg/d.

miconazole nitrate
Micatin, Monistat 3, Monistat 7,
Monistat-Derm

Imidazole derivative; antifungal
PRC: C

Available forms
*Cream, ointment, powder, solution, spray,
vaginal cream:* 2%; *Vaginal suppository:*
100, 200 mg

Indications & dosages
➤ *Tinea pedis, cruris, corporis*—**Adult,
child:** Apply or spray sparingly bid × 2-
4 wk.
➤ *Vulvovaginal candidiasis*—**Adult:** 1 applicator or 100-mg suppository (Monistat
7) inserted intravaginally hs × 7 d; repeat
course prn. Or, 200-mg suppository
(Monistat 3) intravaginally hs × 3 d.

midazolam hydrochloride
Versed

*Benzodiazepine; preop sedative, drug for
conscious sedation, adjunctive treatment
for induction of general anesthesia,
amnestic*
PRC: D; CSS: IV

Available forms
Injection: 1, 5 mg/ml

Indications & dosages
➤ *Preop sedation*—**Adult:** 0.07-0.08 mg/
kg IM 1 hr preop.¶
➤ *Conscious sedation*—**Adult:** 1-2 mg
slow IV injection before procedure.¶

➤ *Induction of general anesthesia*—
Adult: 0.15-0.35 mg/kg over 20-30 sec.
Then, increments of 25% initial dose prn.
Max 0.6 mg/kg. **Unpremedicated adult
≥ 55 yr:** Initially, 0.3 mg/kg.¶

mifepristone
Mifeprex

Synthetic steroid; anti-progestational
PRC: NR

Available forms
Tablets: 200 mg

Indications & dosages
➤ *Termination of intrauterine pregnancy
through 49th d*—**Adult:** 600 mg PO as 1
dose. On d 3, unless abortion is confirmed by clinical exam or ultrasound,
400 mcg misoprostol PO × 1 dose.

miglitol
Glyset

Alpha-glucosidase inhibitor; antidiabetic
PRC: B

Available forms
Tablets: 25, 50, 100 mg

Indications & dosages
➤ *Type 2 DM*—**Adult:** 25 mg PO tid at
start of each main meal; increase prn after
4-8 wk to 50 mg PO tid. May be further
increased after 3 mo based on glycosylat-
ed hemoglobin; max 100 mg PO tid.

milrinone lactate
Primacor

Bipyridine phosphodiesterase inhibitor; inotropic vasodilator
PRC: C

Available forms
Injection: 1 mg/ml; *Injection (premixed):* 200 mcg/ml in D_5W

Indications & dosages
➤ *HF*—**Adult:** Loading dose 50 mcg/kg IV slowly over 10 min; then continue infusion of 0.375-0.75 mcg/kg/min.†

minocycline hydrochloride
Alti-Minocycline*, Apo-Minocycline*, Dynacin, Minocin, Novo-Minocycline*, PMS-Minocycline

Tetracycline; antibiotic
PRC: D

Available forms
Capsules: 50, 75, 100 mg; *Capsules (pellet-filled):* 50, 100 mg; *Injection:* 100 mg/vial; *Tablets:* 50, 75, 100 mg

Indications & dosages
➤ *Infection*—**Adult:** 200 mg IV; then 100 mg IV q 12 hr. Max 400 mg/d. Or, 200 mg PO; then 100 mg PO q 12 hr. Or, 100-200 mg PO; then 50 mg qid.† **Child > 8 yr:** 4 mg/kg PO or IV; then 2 mg/kg q 12 hr IV in 500- to 1,000-ml solution without calcium over 6 hr.†
➤ *Gonorrhea in PCN-allergic patient*— **Adult:** 200 mg PO; then 100 mg q 12 hr ≥ 4 d.†

➤ *Syphilis in PCN-allergic patient*—**Adult:** 200 mg PO; then 100 mg q 12 hr × 10-15 d.†
➤ *Meningococcal carrier state*—**Adult:** 100 mg PO q 12 hr × 5 d.†
➤ *Uncomplicated urethral, endocervical, rectal infection from* Chlamydia trachomatis—100 mg PO q 12 hr × ≥ 7 d.†

minoxidil
Loniten

Peripheral vasodilator; antihypertensive
PRC: C

Available forms
Tablets: 2.5, 10 mg

Indications & dosages
➤ *HTN*—**Adult, child ≥ 12 yr:** 5 mg PO daily. Effective dose 10-40 mg/d. Max 100 mg/d. **Child < 12 yr:** 0.2 mg/kg PO daily; max 5 mg/d. Effective dose 0.25-1 mg/kg/d. Max 50 mg/d.

mirtazapine
Remeron, Remeron SolTab

Piperazinoazepine; tetracyclic antidepressant
PRC: C

Available forms
Tablets: 15, 30, 45 mg; *Tablets (orally disintegrating):* 15, 30, 45 mg

Indications & dosages
Depression—**Adult:** 15 mg PO hs. Maintenance 15-45 mg/d. Adjust dose at ≥ 1-2 wk.

---

misoprostol
Cytotec

Prostaglandin E₁ analogue; antiulcerative, gastric mucosal protectant
PRC: X

Available forms
Tablets: 100, 200 mcg

Indications & dosages
➤ *Prevention of NSAID-induced gastric ulcers*—**Adult:** 200 mcg PO qid (last dose hs) with food; if not tolerated, decrease to 100 mcg PO qid.

moexipril hydrochloride
Univasc

ACE inhibitor; antihypertensive
PRC: C (D, 2nd and 3rd trimesters)

Available forms
Tablets: 7.5, 15 mg

Indications & dosages
➤ *HTN*—**Adult:** 7.5 mg (3.75 mg if patient is on diuretic) PO daily 1 hr ac. Maintenance dose 7.5-30 mg daily, in 1 or 2 divided doses 1 hr ac.†

montelukast sodium
Singulair

Leukotriene receptor antagonist; antiasthmatic
PRC: B

Available forms
Granules: 4-mg packet; *Tablets (chewable):* 4, 5 mg; *Tablets (film-coated):* 10 mg

Indications & dosages
➤ *Asthma, seasonal allergic rhinitis*—**Adult, child ≥ 15 yr:** 10 mg (film-coated) PO daily q pm. **Child 6-14 yr:** 5 mg (chewable) PO daily q pm. **Child 2-5 yr:** 4 mg (chewable) or 1 packet granules PO daily q pm.
➤ *Asthma*—**Child 12-23 mo:** 1 packet of 4-mg granules PO daily q pm.

morphine hydrochloride
Morphitec*, M.O.S.*

morphine sulfate
Astramorph PF, Avinza, Duramorph, Epimorph*, Infumorph 200, Morphine H.P.*, MS Contin, Roxanol

Opioid; opioid analgesic
PRC: C; CSS: II

Available forms
hydrochloride *Oral solution*, syrup*:* 1, 5, 10, 20, 50 mg/ml; *Suppository*:* 10, 20, 30 mg; *Tablets*:* 10, 20, 40, 60 mg; *Tablets (extended-release)*:* 30, 60 mg; **sulfate** *Capsules (extended-release):* 30, 60, 90, 120 mg; *Injection (with preservative):* 0.5, 1, 2, 3, 4, 5, 8, 10, 15, 25, 50 mg/ml; *Injection (without preservative):* 0.5, 1, 10, 25 mg/ml; *Oral solution:* 10, 20, 100 mg/ 5 ml, 20 mg/ml (concentrate); *Solution tablets:* 10, 15, 30 mg; *Suppository:* 5, 10, 20, 30 mg; *Syrup:* 1, 5 mg/ml; *Tablets:* 15,

30 mg; *Tablets (extended-release):* 15, 30,
60, 100, 200 mg

Indications & dosages
➤ *Pain*—**Adult:** 5-20 mg SC or IM, or
2.5-15 mg IV q 4 hr prn; or 10-30 mg PO
or 10-20 mg PR q 4 hr prn. For continuous IV, loading dose 15 mg IV; then infuse
0.8-10 mg/hr. Or, 15-30 mg extended-
release tablet PO q 8-12 hr or 30 mg
extended-release capsule PO daily. Epidural injection, 5 mg; then, if no adequate
pain relief is achieved within 1 hr, additional doses of 1-2 mg. Max total epidural
dose ≤ 10 mg/24 hr. **Child:** 0.1-0.2 mg/kg
SC or IM q 4 hr. Max single dose 15 mg.

moxifloxacin hydrochloride
Avelox, Avelox IV

Fluoroquinolone; antibiotic
PRC: C

Available forms
Infusion: 400 mg/250 ml; *Tablets (film-
coated):* 400 mg

Indications & dosages
➤ *Sinusitis*—**Adult:** 400 mg PO or IV
daily × 10 d.
➤ *Chronic bronchitis exacerbation*—
Adult: 400 mg PO or IV daily × 5 d.
➤ *Community-acquired pneumonia*—
Adult: 400 mg PO or IV daily × 7-14 d.
➤ *Uncomplicated skin and skin-structure
infection*—**Adult:** 400 mg PO or IV daily
× 7 d.

nabumetone
Relafen

NSAID; antarthritic
PRC: C

Available forms
Tablets: 500, 750 mg

Indications & dosages
➤ *RA, OA*—**Adult:** 1,000 mg PO daily in
1 dose or in divided doses bid. Max
2,000 mg/d.

nadolol
Corgard

*Beta blocker; antihypertensive, anti-
anginal*
PRC: C

Available forms
Tablets: 20, 40, 80, 120, 160 mg

Indications & dosages
➤ *Angina*—**Adult:** 40 mg PO daily. Increase by 40-80 mg prn. Maintenance 40-
80 mg/d.†
➤ *HTN*—**Adult:** 40 mg PO daily. Increase by 40-80 mg prn. Maintenance 40-
80 mg/d. Up to 320 mg may be needed.†

nafcillin sodium
Penicillinase-resistant PCN; antibiotic
PRC: B

Available forms
Injection for IV infusion: 1, 2 g

Indications & dosages

➤ *Systemic infections caused by susceptible organisms (methicillin-sensitive* Staphylococcus aureus*)*—**Adult:** 500 mg-1 g IV q 4 hr depending on the severity of the infection. **Infant, child > 1 mo:** 50-200 mg/kg/d IV in divided doses q 4-6 hr depending on the severity of the infection. **Neonate ≤ 7 d, ≤ 2 kg:** 25 mg/kg IV q 12 hr. **Neonate ≤ 7 d, >2 kg:** 25 mg/kg IV q 8 hr. **Neonate > 7 d, ≤ 2 kg:** 25 mg/kg IV q 8 hr. **Neonate > 7 d, > 2 kg:** 25 mg/kg IV q 6 hr.

➤ *Meningitis*—**Adult:** 100-200 mg/kg/d IV in divided doses q 4-6 hr. **Neonate ≤ 7 d, ≤ 2 kg:** 50 mg/kg IV q 12 hr. **Neonate ≤ 7 d, > 2 kg:** 50 mg/kg IV q 8 hr. **Neonate > 7 d, ≤ 2 kg:** 50 mg/kg IV q 8 hr. **Neonate > 7 d, > 2 kg:** 50 mg/kg IV q 6 hr.

➤ *Osteomyelitis*—**Adult:** 1-2 g IV q 4 hr × 4-8 wk. **Infant, child > 1 mo:** 100-200 mg/kg/d in divided doses q 4-6 hr.

➤ *Native valve endocarditis*—**Adult:** 2 g IV q 4 hr × 4-6 wk with gentamicin. **Infant, child > 1 mo:** 100-200 mg/kg/d in divided doses q 4-6 hr.

nalbuphine hydrochloride
Nubain

Opioid agonist-antagonist; opioid partial agonist; analgesic, adjunct to anesthesia
PRC: NR

Available forms
Injection: 10, 20 mg/ml

Indications & dosages

➤ *Pain*—**Adult:** Typical (70-kg) patient, 10-20 mg SC, IM, or IV q 3-6 hr prn. Max 160 mg/d.

➤ *Adjunct to anesthesia*—**Adult:** 0.3-3 mg/kg IV over 10-15 min; then maintenance dose 0.25-0.5 mg/kg IV prn.

naloxone hydrochloride
Narcan

Opioid antagonist; opioid antagonist
PRC: B

Available forms
Injection: 0.02, 0.4, 1 mg/ml

Indications & dosages

➤ *Opioid-induced respiratory depression*—**Adult:** 0.4-2 mg IV, SC, or IM. Repeat q 2-3 min prn. Reconsider diagnosis if no response after 10 mg. **Child:** 0.01 mg/kg IV; then 2nd dose of 0.1 mg/kg IV prn. If no IV, give IM or SC in divided doses. **Neonate:** 0.01 mg/kg IV, IM, or SC. Repeat dose q 2-3 min prn.

➤ *Postop opioid depression*—**Adult:** 0.1-0.2 mg IV q 2-3 min until desired degree of reversal is reached. Repeat dose within 1-2 hr if needed. **Child:** 0.005-0.01 mg IV. Repeat q 2-3 min until desired degree of reversal is reached.

➤ *Opiate-induced asphyxia neonatorum*—**Neonate:** 0.01 mg/kg IV via umbilical vein. Repeat q 2-3 min until desired degree of reversal is reached.

---

§ Adjust in immunocompromised patients   ¶ Adjust in debilitated patients

naltrexone hydrochloride
Depade, ReVia

Opioid antagonist; opioid detoxification adjunct
PRC: C

Available forms
Tablets: 50 mg

Indications & dosages
➤ *Maintenance of opioid-free state in detoxified patient*—**Adult:** 25 mg PO. If no withdrawal signs after 1 hr, give additional 25 mg. When patient is using 50 mg q 24 hr, use flexible maintenance schedule.
➤ *Alcohol dependence*—**Adult:** 50 mg PO daily.

naproxen
EC-Naprosyn, Naprosyn, Naprosyn SR*, Novo-Naprox*

naproxen sodium
Aleve, Anaprox, Apo-Napro-Na*, Naprelan, Synflex*

NSAID; nonopioid analgesic, antipyretic, anti-inflammatory
PRC: B

Available forms
naproxen *Oral suspension:* 125 mg/5 ml; *Tablets:* 250, 375, 500 mg; *Tablets (delayed-release):* 375, 500 mg; *Tablets (extended-release):* 750, 1,000 mg; **sodium** *Tablets (controlled-release):* 421.5, 550 mg; *Tablets (film-coated):* 220, 275, 550 mg. *Note:* 275 mg naproxen sodium = 250 mg naproxen

Indications & dosages
➤ *RA, OA, ankylosing spondylitis, pain, dysmenorrhea, tendinitis, bursitis*—
Adult: 250-500 mg (naproxen) bid; max 1.5 g/d. Or, 375-500 mg delayed-release (EC-Naprosyn) bid; or 750-1,000 mg controlled-release (Naprelan) bid; or 275-550 mg sodium bid.
➤ *Juvenile arthritis*—**Child:** 10 mg/kg PO in 2 divided doses.
➤ *Gout*—**Adult:** 750 mg (naproxen) PO, then 250 mg q 8 hr until attack subsides. Or, 825 mg sodium, then 275 mg q 8 hr until attack subsides; or 1,000-1,500 mg/d controlled-release (Naprelan) on 1st d, then 1,000 mg/d.
➤ *Pain*—**Adult:** 500 mg (naproxen) PO, then 250 mg q 6-8 hr, max 1.25 g/d. Or, 550 mg sodium, then 275 mg q 6-8 hr, max 1.375 g/d; or 1,000 mg controlled-release (Naprelan) daily.

nateglinide
Starlix

Amino acid derivative; antidiabetic
PRC: C

Available forms
Tablets: 60, 120 mg

Indications & dosages
➤ *Alone or with metformin, to treat hyperglycemia in patient with type 2 DM*—
Adult: 120 mg PO tid, ≤ 30 min ac. If HbA_{1c} is near goal when treatment starts, 60 mg PO tid.

---

nefazodone hydrochloride
Serzone

Phenylpiperazine; antidepressant
PRC: C

Available forms
Tablets: 100, 150, 200, 250 mg

Indications & dosages
➤ *Depression*—**Adult:** 200 mg/d PO in 2 divided doses.¶ Increase 100-200 mg/d at ≥ 1 wk prn. Range 300-600 mg/d. **Elderly:** 50 mg PO bid.

nelfinavir mesylate
Viracept

HIV protease inhibitor; antiviral
PRC: B

Available forms
Powder: 50 mg/g powder in 144-g bottle; *Tablets:* 250, 625 mg

Indications & dosages
➤ *HIV infection*—**Adult:** 750 mg PO tid. Or, 1,250 mg PO bid with meal. **Child 2-13 yr:** 20-30 mg/kg PO tid. Max 750 mg PO tid.

neostigmine bromide
Prostigmin

neostigmine methylsulfate
Prostigmin

Cholinesterase inhibitor; muscle stimulant
PRC: C

Available forms
bromide *Tablets:* 15 mg; **methylsulfate** *Injection:* 0.25, 0.5, 1 mg/ml

Indications & dosages
➤ *Myasthenia gravis*—**Adult:** 0.5 mg SC or IM. Or, 15-375 mg/d PO. **Child:** 7.5-15 mg PO tid or qid.
➤ *Diagnosis of myasthenia gravis*—**Adult:** 0.022 mg/kg IM 30 min after atropine IM. **Child:** 0.025-0.04 mg/kg IM after atropine SC.
➤ *Postop abdominal distention and bladder atony*—**Adult:** 0.5-1 mg IM or SC q 3 hr × 5 doses after bladder is emptied.
➤ *Antidote for nondepolarizing neuromuscular blockers*—**Adult:** 0.5-2 mg IV slowly. Repeat prn. Max 5 mg. Before antidote dose, give atropine IV.

nesiritide
Natrecor

Human B-type natriuretic peptide; inotropic vasodilator
PRC: C

Available forms
Injection: Single-dose vials 1.5 mg sterile, lyophilized powder

Indications & dosages
➤ *Acutely decompensated and symptomatic HF*—**Adult:** 2 mcg/kg IV over 60 sec; then continue infusion of 0.01 mcg/kg/min.

---

§ Adjust in immunocompromised patients   ¶ Adjust in debilitated patients

nevirapine
Viramune

Nonnucleoside reverse transcriptase inhibitor; antiviral
PRC: C

Available forms
PO suspension: 50 mg/5 ml; *Tablets:* 200 mg

Indications & dosages
➤ *HIV-1 infection*—**Adult:** 200 mg PO daily × 1st 14 d, then 200 mg PO bid. **Child ≥ 8 yr:** 4 mg/kg PO daily × 14 d, then 4 mg/kg PO bid. Max 400 mg/d. **Child 2 mo-8 yr:** 4 mg/kg PO daily × 14 d, then 7 mg/kg PO bid. Max 400 mg/d.

niacin (nicotinic acid, vitamin B₃)
Niac, Niacor, Nico-400, Nicobid, Nicolar

niacinamide (nicotinamide)

B-complex vitamin; vitamin B₃, antilipemic, peripheral vasodilator
PRC: C

Available forms
niacin *Capsules (timed-release):* 125, 250, 300, 400, 500 mg; *Elixir:* 50 mg/5 ml; *Injection:* 100 mg/ml in 30-ml vials; *Tablets:* 25, 50, 100, 250, 500 mg; *Tablets (timed-release):* 250, 375, 500, 750, 1,000 mg; **niacinamide** *Tablets:* 50, 100, 125, 250, 500 mg

Indications & dosages
➤ *Pellagra*—**Adult:** 300-500 mg PO, SC, IM, or IV daily in divided doses. **Child:** Up to 300 mg PO daily in divided doses.
➤ *Hyperlipidemia (niacin only)*—**Adult:** 1-2 g PO tid with meals or pc; may increase to 6 g/d.

nicardipine
Cardene, Cardene I.V., Cardene SR

Calcium channel blocker; antianginal, antihypertensive
PRC: C

Available forms
Capsules (immediate-release): 20, 30 mg; *Capsules (sustained-release):* 30, 45, 60 mg; *Injection:* 2.5 mg/ml

Indications & dosages
➤ *Angina, HTN*—**Adult:** 20 mg PO tid (immediate-release). Adjust to response q 3 d. Range 20-40 mg tid. Range 30-60 mg (sustained-release) bid.
➤ *HTN (short-term)*—**Adult:** If unable to take PO nicardipine, 5 mg/hr IV; titrate to 2.5 mg/hr q 15 min; max 15 mg/hr.

nicotine transdermal system
Habitrol, Nicoderm, Nicotrol

Nicotinic cholinergic agonist; smoking cessation aid
PRC: D

Available forms
Habitrol, Nicoderm: 7, 14, 21 mg/d; *Nicotrol:* 5, 10, 15 mg/16 hr

---

Indications & dosages

➤ *Smoking cessation*—**Adult:** 1 system, delivering largest available nicotine dose in series, applied daily. For Habitrol and Nicoderm, patch is kept on 24 hr, then removed and new system applied to alternate skin site. For Nicotrol, patch is applied in am and removed hs. After 4-12 wk, taper to next lowest dose in series; then in 2-4 wk, to lowest system in series. Stop in 2-4 wk.

nifedipine
Adalat, Adalat CC, Apo-Nifed*, Nifedical XL, Nu-Nifed*, Procardia, Procardia XL

Calcium channel blocker; antianginal, antihypertensive
PRC: C

Available forms

Capsules: 10, 20 mg; *Tablets (extended-release):* 30, 60, 90 mg

Indications & dosages

➤ *Prinzmetal's angina*—**Adult:** 10 mg PO tid. Range 10-20 mg tid. Max 180 mg/d.
➤ *HTN*—**Adult:** 30 or 60 mg PO daily. Adjust over 7-14 d. Doses > 90 mg (for Adalat CC) and > 120 mg (for Procardia XL, Nifedical XL) not recommended.

nisoldipine
Sular

Calcium channel blocker; antihypertensive
PRC: C

Available forms

Tablets (extended-release): 10, 20, 30, 40 mg

Indications & dosages

➤ *HTN*—**Adult:** 20 mg PO daily‡; increase by 10 mg/wk or at longer intervals prn. Maintenance 20-40 mg/d. Max 60 mg/d. **Elderly:** Initially ≤ 10 mg PO daily.

nitazoxanide
Alinia, Cryptaz

Antiprotozoan; antidiarrheal, anti-infective
PRC: B

Available forms

Powder for injection: 100 mg/5 ml in 60-ml bottle

Indications & dosages

➤ *Diarrhea caused by* Cryptosporidium parvum *and* Giardia lamblia—**Child 12-47 mo:** 5 ml (100 mg) PO q 12 hr × 3 d with food. **Child 4-11 yr:** 10 ml (200 mg) PO q 12 hr × 3 d with food.

nitrofurantoin macrocrystals
Macrobid, Macrodantin

nitrofurantoin microcrystals
Furadantin

Nitrofuran; urinary tract anti-infective
PRC: B

---

§ Adjust in immunocompromised patients   ¶ Adjust in debilitated patients

Available forms
macrocrystals *Capsules:* 25, 50, 100 mg;
microcrystals *Oral suspension:* 25 mg/
5 ml

Indications & dosages
➤ *UTI*—**Adult, child > 12 yr:** 50-100 mg
PO qid with meals and hs. Or, 100 mg
Macrobid PO q 12 hr × 7 d. **Child 1 mo-
12 yr:** 5-7 mg/kg PO daily divided qid.
➤ *Suppression treatment*—**Adult:** 50-
100 mg PO q hs. **Child:** 1 mg/kg PO daily
in 1 dose hs or divided into 2 doses.

nitroglycerin (glyceryl trinitrate)
Nitro-Bid, Nitrocine, Nitrodisc,
Nitro-Dur, Nitrogard, Nitroglyn, Nitrol,
Nitrolingual, Nitrostat, Transderm-Nitro,
Tridil

Nitrate; antianginal, vasodilator
PRC: C

Available forms
Aerosol (translingual): 0.4-mg metered
spray; *Capsules (sustained-release):* 2.5,
6.5, 9, 13 mg; *Injection:* 0.5, 5 mg/ml;
Tablets (buccal): 1, 2, 3 mg; *Tablets (SL):*
0.3, 0.4, 0.6 mg; *Tablets (sustained-
release):* 2.6, 6.5, 9, 13 mg; *Topical ointment:* 2%; *Transdermal:* 0.1, 0.2, 0.3, 0.4,
0.6, 0.8 mg/hr release rate

Indications & dosages
➤ *Angina prophylaxis*—**Adult:** 2.5 mg or
2.6 mg sustained-release capsule q 8-
12 hr. Or, 2% ointment, ½-5 inches. Or,
transdermal disc or pad 0.2-0.4 mg/hr
daily.

➤ *Acute angina, angina prophylaxis*—
Adult: 1 SL tablet. Repeat q 5 min prn, ×
15 min. Or, use Nitrolingual, 1 or 2 sprays
into mouth. Repeat q 3-5 min prn, to max
3 doses in 15 min. Or, 1-3 mg transmu-
cosally q 3-5 hr while awake.
➤ *HTN, HF, angina, control HTN during
surgery, produce controlled hypotension
during surgery*—**Adult:** 5 mcg/min; increase prn by 5 mcg/min q 3-5 min until
response.

nitroprusside sodium
Nitropress

Vasodilator; antihypertensive
PRC: C

Available forms
Injection: 50 mg/vial in 2-, 5-ml vials

Indications & dosages
➤ *HTN emergencies*—**Adult, child:**
50-mg vial diluted with 2-3 ml D₅W and
added to 250, 500, or 1,000 ml D₅W; infuse at 0.3-10 mcg/kg/min titrated to BP.
Max rate 10 mcg/kg/min.
➤ *HF*—**Adult, child:** IV infusion titrated
to cardiac output and BP. Same dose
range as for HTN emergencies.

nizatidine
Axid, Axid AR

H₂-receptor antagonist; antiulcerative
PRC: C

Available forms
Capsules: 150, 300 mg

Indications & dosages
➤ *Active duodenal ulcer*—**Adult:** 300 mg PO daily hs. Or, 150 mg PO bid.
➤ *Maintenance for duodenal ulcer*—**Adult:** 150 mg PO daily hs.
➤ *Benign gastric ulcer*—**Adult:** 150 mg PO bid or 300 mg hs × 8 wk.
➤ *GERD*—**Adult:** 150 mg PO bid.

norepinephrine bitartrate
Levophed

Adrenergic; vasopressor
PRC: C

Available forms
Injection: 1 mg/ml

Indications & dosages
➤ *Acute hypotension*—**Adult:** 8-12 mcg/min IV infusion, titrate to maintain normal BP. Maintenance 2-4 mcg/min. **Child:** 2 mcg/m²/min IV infusion. Titrate prn.

norethindrone
Camilla, Errin, Micronor, Nora-BE, Nor-QD

norethindrone acetate
Aygestin, Norlutate

Progestin; hormonal contraceptive
PRC: X

Available forms
norethindrone *Tablets:* 0.35 mg; **acetate** *Tablets:* 5 mg

Indications & dosages
➤ *Amenorrhea, abnormal uterine bleeding*—**Adult:** 2.5-20 mg PO daily on d 5-25 of menstrual cycle.
➤ *Endometriosis*—**Adult:** 5-10 mg PO daily × 14 d; then increase by 2.5-5 mg/d q 2 wk up to 15 mg/d.
➤ *Contraception*—**Adult:** 0.35 mg norethindrone PO on d 1 of menstruation; then 0.35 mg/d.

nortriptyline hydrochloride
Aventyl, Pamelor

TCA; antidepressant
PRC: NR

Available forms
Capsules: 10, 25, 50, 75 mg; *Oral solution:* 10 mg/5 ml (4% alcohol)

Indications & dosages
➤ *Depression*—**Adult:** 25 mg PO tid or qid, increase to max 150 mg/d. Entire dose may be given hs. Monitor plasma levels for doses > 100 mg/d. **Elderly:** 30-50 mg PO daily in 1 dose or 2 divided doses.

nystatin
Mycostatin, Nadostine*, Nilstat, Nystex

Polyene macrolide; antifungal
PRC: C

Available forms
Cream, ointment, powder: 100,000 units/g; *Lozenges:* 200,000 units; *Oral suspension:* 100,000 units/ml; 50, 150, 500 million units; 1, 2 billion units; *Tablets:* 500,000

units; *Troche:* 200,000 units; *Vaginal tablets:* 100,000 units

Indications & dosages

➤ *Intestinal candidiasis*—**Adult:** 500,000-1 million units as PO tablet tid.
➤ *Oral infection*—**Adult, child:** 400,000-600,000 units oral suspension qid. **Infant:** 200,000 units oral suspension qid. **Neonate, premature infant:** 100,000 units oral suspension qid.
➤ *Vaginal yeast infection*—**Adult:** 100,000 units (tablet) high into vagina daily × 14 d.

ofloxacin
Floxin

Fluoroquinolone; antibiotic
PRC: C

Available forms

Tablets (film-coated): 200, 300, 400 mg

Indications & dosages

➤ *Lower respiratory tract infection*—**Adult:** 400 mg PO q 12 hr × 10 d.†
➤ *Cervicitis, urethritis*—**Adult:** 300 mg PO q 12 hr × 7 d.†
➤ *Gonorrhea*—**Adult:** 400 mg PO in 1 dose with doxycycline.†
➤ *Skin infection*—**Adult:** 400 mg PO q 12 hr × 10 d.†
➤ *Cystitis, UTI*—**Adult:** 200 mg PO q 12 hr × 3-7 d.†
➤ *Prostatitis*—**Adult:** 300 mg PO q 12 hr × 6 wk.†
➤ *PID (outpatient)*—**Adult:** 400 mg PO q 12 hr × 14 d.†

olanzapine
Zyprexa, Zyprexa Zydis

Dibenzapine derivative; antipsychotic
PRC: C

Available forms

Tablets: 2.5, 5, 7.5, 10, 15, 20 mg; *Tablets (orally disintegrating):* 5, 10, 15, 20 mg

Indications & dosages

➤ *Acute mania (bipolar I disorder)*—**Adult:** 10-15 mg PO daily. Adjust dose 5 mg/d at intervals of ≥ 24 hr prn. Max 20 mg/d. Duration of treatment is 3-4 wk.¶
➤ *Schizophrenia*—**Adult:** 5-10 mg PO daily. Adjust dose 5 mg/d at intervals of ≥ 1 wk. Target dose of 10 mg/d. Max 20 mg/d.¶
Note: The recommended starting dose is 5 mg PO in patients predisposed to hypotensive reactions, in those who have risk factors of slower metabolism of olanzapine (nonsmoking female patients > 65), or in those who are pharmacodynamically sensitive to olanzapine. Adjust dose cautiously in these patients.

olmesartan medoxomil
Benicar

Angiotensin II receptor antagonist; antihypertensive
PRC: C (first trimester) and D (second and third trimesters)

Available forms

Tablets: 5, 20, 40 mg

Indications & dosages

➤ *HTN*—**Adult:** 20 mg PO daily in patients who aren't volume-contracted. May increase dose to 40 mg PO daily if BP isn't reduced after 2 wk of therapy.†

omeprazole
Losec*, Prilosec

Proton pump inhibitor; gastric acid suppressant
PRC: C

Available forms
Capsules (delayed-release): 10, 20, 40 mg

Indications & dosages

➤ *Esophagitis, GERD*—**Adult:** 20 mg PO daily × 4-8 wk.‡
➤ *Hypersecretory conditions*—**Adult:** 60 mg PO daily; adjust to response. If dose > 80 mg, give in divided doses.‡
➤ *Duodenal ulcer*—**Adult:** 20 mg PO daily × 4-8 wk.‡
➤ *Active benign gastric ulcer*—**Adult:** 40 mg PO daily × 4-8 wk.‡
➤ *Helicobacter pylori infection*—**Adult:** 40 mg PO q am with clarithromycin × 14 d; then 20 mg daily × 14 d.‡

ondansetron hydrochloride
Zofran, Zofran ODT

Serotonin (5-HT$_3$) receptor antagonist; antiemetic
PRC: B

Available forms
Injection: 2 mg/ml; *Oral solution:* 4 mg/5 ml; *Premixed injection:* 32 mg/50 ml;

Tablets: 4, 8, 24 mg; *Tablets (orally disintegrating):* 4, 8 mg

Indications & dosages

➤ *Nausea, vomiting with chemo*—**Adult, child ≥ 12 yr:** 8 mg PO 30 min before chemo. Then, 8 mg PO 8 hr after 1st dose, then 8 mg q 12 hr × 1-2 d. Or, 1 dose of 32 mg/15 ml IV 30 min before chemo; or 3 divided doses of 0.15 mg/kg IV over 15 min, 4 and 8 hr after 1st dose (30 min before chemo).‡ **Child 4-12 yr:** 4 mg PO 30 min before chemo. Then 4 mg PO 4 and 8 hr after 1st dose, then 4 mg q 8 hr × 1-2 d. Or, 3 doses of 0.15 mg/kg IV, as for adult.‡
➤ *Prevention of nausea, vomiting with highly emetogenic chemo*—**Adult:** 24 mg PO 30 min before administration of single-day chemo.‡
➤ *Nausea, vomiting with radiation*—**Adult:** 8 mg PO tid.‡

oseltamivir phosphate
Tamiflu

Neuraminidase inhibitor; antiviral
PRC: C

Available forms
Capsules: 75 mg; *Oral suspension:* 12 mg/ml

Indications & dosages

➤ *Symptomatic influenza ≤ 2 d*—**Adult, child ≥ 13 yr:** 75 mg PO bid × 5 d.†
➤ *Prevention of influenza after close contact with infected person*—**Adult, child ≥ 13 yr:** 75 mg PO daily within 2 d of exposure and lasting ≥ 7 d.†

§ Adjust in immunocompromised patients   ¶ Adjust in debilitated patients

▶ *Prevention of influenza during community outbreak*—**Adult, child ≥ 13 yr:** 75 mg PO daily × ≤ 6 wk.†
▶ *Influenza*—**Child ≥ 1 yr: ≤ 15 kg:** 30 mg oral suspension PO bid.† **> 15-23 kg:** 45 mg oral suspension PO bid.† **> 23-40 kg:** 60 mg oral suspension PO bid.† **> 40 kg:** 75 mg oral suspension PO bid.†

oxaliplatin
Eloxatin

Alkylating drug; antineoplastic
PRC: D

Available forms
Injection: 50- or 100-mg vials

Indications & dosages
▶ *Metastatic colon or rectal cancer that has recurred or progressed during or within 6 mo of completion of 1st-line therapy with 5-fluorouracil (5-FU)/, leucovorin, and irinotecan*—**Adult: Day 1:** 85 mg/m² oxaliplatin IV in 250 to 500 ml D₅W and leucovorin 200 mg/m² IV in D₅W, given simultaneously over 120 min, in separate bags using a Y-line, followed by 5-FU 400 mg/m² IV bolus over 2 to 4 min, followed by 600 mg/m² 5-FU IV infusion in 500 ml D₅W over 22 hr. **Day 2:** 200 mg/m² leucovorin IV infusion over 120 min, followed by 400 mg/m² 5-FU IV bolus over 2 to 4 min, followed by 600 mg/m² 5-FU IV infusion in 500 ml D₅W over 22 hr. Repeat cycle q 2 wk. **Patients with unresolved and persistent grade 2 neurosensory events:** Reduce dose to 65 mg/m². **Patients with persist-**

ent grade 3 neurosensory events: Consider stopping drug. **Patients recovering from grade 3 or 4 GI or hematologic events:** Reduce dose to 65 mg/m². Also reduce dose of 5-FU by 20%.

oxazepam
Apo-Oxazepam*, Novoxapam*, Serax

Benzodiazepine; anxiolytic, sedative-hypnotic
PRC: NR; CSS: IV

Available forms
Capsules: 10, 15, 30 mg; *Tablets:* 15 mg

Indications & dosages
▶ *Alcohol withdrawal, severe anxiety*—**Adult:** 15-30 mg PO tid or qid.
▶ *Anxiety*—**Adult:** 10-15 mg PO tid or qid. **Elderly:** 10 mg tid, increase to 15 mg tid or qid prn.

oxcarbazepine
Trileptel

Carboxamide derivative; antiepileptic
PRC: C

Available forms
Oral suspension: 60 mg/ml; 300 mg/5 ml; *Tablets (film-coated):* 150, 300, 600 mg

Indications & dosages
▶ *Adjunct treatment for partial seizures*—**Adult:** 300 mg PO bid. Increase by max 600 mg/d q wk. Recommended dose 1,200 mg/d divided bid. **Child 4-16 yr:** Initially 8-10 mg/kg/d PO divided bid, not > 600 mg/d. Target maintenance

dose is divided bid reached over 2 wk. If patient 20-29 kg, target maintenance dose is 900 mg/d. If patient > 29-39 kg, target maintenance dose is 1,200 mg/d. If patient > 39 kg, target maintenance dose is 1,800 mg/d.†

➤ *Conversion to monotherapy for treatment of partial seizures*—**Adult:** 300 mg PO bid while simultaneously reducing the dose of other antiepileptics over 3-6 wk until they are completely withdrawn. Increase oxcarbazepine by max 600 mg/d q wk over 2-4 wk to 2,400 mg/d divided bid.†

➤ *Monotherapy partial seizures*—**Adult:** 300 mg PO bid. Increase by 300 mg/d q 3 d to 1,200 mg/d divided bid.†

oxycodone hydrochloride
OxyContin, OxyFAST, Oxy IR, Roxicodone, Roxicodone Intensol, Supeudol*

Opioid; analgesic
PRC: B; CSS: II

Available forms
Capsules (immediate-release): 5 mg; *Oral solution:* 5, 20 mg/ml (concentrate); *Suppository***:* 10, 20 mg; *Tablets:* 5 mg; *Tablets (controlled-release):* 10, 20, 40, 80 mg; *Tablets (immediate-release):* 15, 30 mg

Indications & dosages
➤ *Pain*—**Adult:** 10-30 mg PO q 4 hr (5 mg PO q 6 hr for Oxy IR, OxyFAST, and immediate-release capsules). Or, 10-40 mg PR tid or qid. Or, 10 mg controlled-release q 12 hr initially in opioid-naive patients.

oxytocin, synthetic injection
Pitocin

Exogenous hormone; oxytocic, lactation stimulant
PRC: NR

Available forms
Injection: 10 units/ampule, vial, syringe

Indications & dosages
➤ *Induction, stimulation of labor*—**Adult:** 1-ml (10 units) ampule in 1,000 ml D₅W or NSS IV infusion at 1-2 milliunits/min. Increase in increments of ≤ 1-2 milliunits/min q 15-30 min.
➤ *Postpartum bleeding*—**Adult:** 10-40 units added to 1 L D₅W or NSS infusion at 20-40 milliunits/min; 1 ml (10 units) may be given IM after placenta delivery.
➤ *Incomplete or inevitable abortion*—**Adult:** 10 units IV in 500 ml NSS or D₅NSS at 10-20 milliunits/min.

paclitaxel
Taxol

Antimicrotubule agent; antineoplastic
PRC: D

Available forms
Injection: 30 mg/5 ml, 100 mg/16.7 ml

Indications & dosages
➤ *Advanced ovarian CA*—**Adult (previously untreated):** 175 mg/m² IV over 3 hr q 3 wk followed by cisplatin 75 mg/m²; or, 135 mg/m² IV over 24 hr with cisplatin 75 mg/m² q 3 wk. Don't repeat until neu-

§ Adjust in immunocompromised patients   ¶ Adjust in debilitated patients

trophil count ≥ 1,500 cells/mm³ and platelet count ≥ 100,000 cells/mm³.‡ **Adult (previously treated):** 135 or 175 mg/m² IV over 3 hr q 3 wk. Don't repeat until neutrophil count ≥ 1,500 cells/mm³ and platelet count ≥ 100,000 cells/mm³.‡

➤ *Breast CA after failure of combination chemo for metastatic disease or relapse within 6 mo of adjuvant chemo (prior treatment should have included an anthracycline unless contraindicated); adjuvant treatment of node-positive breast CA administered sequentially to standard doxorubicin-containing combination chemotherapy*—**Adult:** 175 mg/m² IV over 3 hr q 3 wk. Don't repeat until neutrophil count ≥ 1,500 cells/mm³ and platelet count ≥ 100,000 cells/mm³.‡

➤ *AIDS-related Kaposi's sarcoma*—**Adult:** 135 mg/m² IV over 3 hr q 3 wk or 100 mg/m² IV over 3 hr q 2 wk. Don't repeat until neutrophil count ≥ 1,000 cells/mm³.‡

➤ *Initial treatment of advanced non-small cell lung CA for patient who isn't candidate for curative surgery or radiation*—**Adult:** 135 mg/m² IV over 24 hr or 175 mg/m² IV over 3 hr. Follow with cisplatin 75 mg/m² or 80 mg/m², respectively. Repeat q 3 wk. Don't repeat until neutrophil count ≥ 1,500 cells/mm³ and platelet count ≥ 100,000 cells/mm³.‡

pamidronate disodium
Aredia

Diphosphonate, pyrophosphate analogue; antihypercalcemic
PRC: D

Available forms
Injection: 30-, 60-, 90-mg vials

Indications & dosages
➤ *Hypercalcemia in CA*—**Patient with albumin-corrected serum calcium (CCa) 12-13.5 mg/dl:** 60-90 mg IV over 2-24 hr. **Patient with CCa > 13.5 mg/dl:** 90 mg IV over 24 hr ≥ 7 d before retreatment.†
➤ *Paget's disease*—**Adult:** 30 mg IV over 4 hr × 3 d. Repeat prn.†
➤ *Osteolytic bone lesions of multiple myeloma*—**Adult:** 90 mg IV over 4 hr q 4 wk.†
➤ *Osteolytic bone lesions of breast CA*—**Adult:** 90 mg IV over 2 hr q 3-4 wk.†

pantoprazole sodium
Protonix, Protonix I.V.

Substituted benzimidazole; gastric acid suppressant
PRC: B

Available forms
Injection: 40 mg; *Tablets (delayed-release):* 20, 40 mg

Indications & dosages
➤ *Esophagitis from GERD*—**Adult:** 40 mg PO daily for ≤ 8 wk; continue another 8 wk prn. If oral therapy is interrupted, may give 40 mg IV daily × 7-10 d.
➤ *Short-term treatment of GERD associated with history of erosive esophagitis*—**Adult:** 40 mg IV daily × 7-10 d. Switch to PO form when tolerated.
➤ *Long-term maintenance of healing erosive esophagitis in patients with GERD*—**Adult:** 40 mg PO daily.

➤ *Pathological hypersecretory conditions, including Zollinger-Ellison syndrome*—**Adult:** Individualize dosage. For short-term treatment, usual dose is 80 mg IV q 12 hr. For those needing a higher dose, 80 mg q 8 hr is expected to maintain acid output less than 10 mEq/hr. Max 240 mg/d. For long-term treatment, usual starting dose is 40 mg PO bid. Max 240 mg/d.

paroxetine hydrochloride
Paxil, Paxil CR

SSRI; antidepressant
PRC: C

Available forms
Oral suspension: 10 mg/5 ml; *Tablets:* 10, 20, 30, 40 mg; *Tablets (controlled-release):* 12.5, 25, 37.5 mg

Indications & dosages
➤ *Depression*—**Adult:** 20 mg PO q am. Increase by 10 mg/d at intervals of 1 wk prn to max 50 mg daily. Or, give 25 mg/d (controlled-release); increase prn by 12.5 mg at intervals of at least 1 wk; max 62.5 mg/d.¶ **Elderly:** 10 mg PO q am. Increase 10 mg/d at intervals of 1 wk prn to max 40 mg daily. Or, 12.5 mg/d (controlled-release); may increase prn to max 50 mg/d.†,‡,¶
➤ *Generalized anxiety disorders, post-traumatic stress disorder*—**Adult:** 20 mg PO daily. Increase by 10 mg/d q wk. Max 50 mg/d.†,‡
➤ *Panic disorder*—**Adult:** 10 mg/d. Increase 10 mg/wk prn. Max 60 mg/d. Or, 12.5 mg PO daily (controlled-release);

may increase prn by 12.5 mg/wk to max 75 mg/d.†,‡ **Elderly:** 10 mg PO daily. Increase prn to max 40 mg/d. Or, 12.5 mg/day (controlled-release); may increase prn to max 50 mg/d.†,‡,¶
➤ *OCD, social anxiety disorder*—**Adult:** 20 mg PO daily in am. Range 20-60 mg/d.†,‡ **Elderly:** 10 mg PO daily. Increase prn; max 40 mg/d.†,‡,¶

pegfilgrastim
Neulasta

Colony-stimulating factor; neutrophil-growth stimulator
PRC: C

Available forms
Injection: 6 mg/0.6 ml syringes

Indications & dosages
➤ *Prevent infection during myelosuppressive anticancer therapy for non-myeloid malignancies*—**Adult:** 6 mg SC once/chemo cycle. Don't give 14 d before to 24 hr after cytotoxic chemo.

peginterferon alfa-2a
Pegasys

Biological response modifier; antiviral
PRC: C

Available forms
Injection: 180 mcg/1 ml

Indications & dosages
➤ *Chronic hepatitis C with compensated hepatic disease in patients not previously treated with interferon alfa*—**Adult:**

---

§ Adjust in immunocompromised patients　　　　　　　　¶ Adjust in debilitated patients

180 mcg SC in abdomen or thigh q wk × 48 wk. **Patients with moderate adverse reactions:** Decrease to 135 mcg SC q wk. **Patients with severe adverse reactions:** Decrease to 90 mcg SC q wk. **Patients with hematological reactions and neutrophil count (ANC) < 750 cells/mm³:** Reduce dose to 135 mcg SC q wk. **Patients with hematological reactions and absolute neutrophil count (ANC) < 500 cells/mm³:** Stop drug until ANC > 1,000 cells/mm³; restart at 90 mcg SC q wk. If platelet count is < 50,000 cells/mm³, reduce dose to 90 mcg SC q wk; stop drug if platelet count goes below 25,000 cells/mm³.†,‡

penicillin G benzathine
Bicillin L-A, Permapen

Natural PCN; antibiotic
PRC: B

Available forms
Injection: 300,000, 600,000 units/ml; 1,200,000 units/2 ml; 2,400,000 units/4 ml

Indications & dosages
➤ *Congenital syphilis*—**Child < 2 yr:** 50,000 units/kg IM × 1 dose.
➤ *Group A strep upper respiratory tract infection*—**Adult:** 1.2 million units IM × 1 dose. **Older child ≥ 27 kg:** 900,000 units IM × 1 dose. **Infant, child < 27 kg:** 300,000-600,000 units IM × 1 dose.
➤ *Prophylaxis of post-strep rheumatic fever*—**Adult, child:** 1.2 million units IM q mo or 600,000 units 2 times/mo.
➤ *Syphilis*—**Adult:** 2.4 million units IM × 1 dose (if duration of infection < 1 yr); or, q wk × 3 wk (if duration of infection > 1 yr).

penicillin G potassium
Pfizerpen

Natural PCN; antibiotic
PRC: B

Available forms
Injection: 1, 5, 10, 20 million units

Indications & dosages
➤ *Systemic infection*—**Adult, child ≥ 12 yr:** 1.2-24 million units IM or IV daily in divided doses q 4 hr.† **Child < 12 yr:** 25,000-400,000 units/kg IM or IV daily in divided doses q 4 hr.†
➤ *Anthrax*—**Adult:** 5-20 million units IV daily in divided doses q 4-6 hr × ≥ 14 d after symptoms abate.† **Child:** 100,000-150,000 units/kg/d IV in divided doses q 4-6 hr × ≥ 14 d after symptoms abate.†

penicillin G procaine

Natural PCN; antibiotic
PRC: B

Available forms
Injection: 600,000, 1,200,000 units/ml

Indications & dosages
➤ *Systemic infection*—**Adult:** 600,000-1.2 million units IM daily in 1 dose. **Child > 1 mo:** 25,000-50,000 units/kg IM daily in 1 dose.
➤ *Gonorrhea*—**Adult, child > 12 yr:** 1 g probenecid PO; after 30 min, 4.8 million units IM, divided between 2 sites.
➤ *Pneumococcal pneumonia*—**Adult, child > 12 yr:** 600,000-1.2 million units IM daily × 7-10 d.

➤ *Anthrax, including inhalation anthrax (post-exposure)*—**Adult:** 1.2 million units IM q 12 hr. **Child:** 25,000 units/kg IM (max 1,200,000 units) q 12 hr.
➤ *Cutaneous anthrax*—**Adult:** 600,000-1 million units IM daily.

penicillin G sodium
Crystapen*

Natural PCN; antibiotic
PRC: B

Available forms
Injection: 5 million–unit vial

Indications & dosages
➤ *Systemic infection*—**Adult, child ≥ 12 yr:** 1.2-24 million units daily IM or IV in divided doses q 4-6 hr.† **Child < 12 yr:** 25,000-400,000 units/kg IM or IV in divided doses q 4-6 hr.†

pentoxifylline
Trental

Xanthine derivative; hemorheologic
PRC: C

Available forms
Tablets (controlled-release): 400 mg; *Tablets (extended-release):* 400 mg

Indications & dosages
➤ *Intermittent claudication*—**Adult:** 400 mg PO tid with meals. May decrease to 400 mg bid if adverse reactions occur.

pergolide mesylate
Permax

Dopaminergic agonist; antiparkinsonian
PRC: B

Available forms
Tablets: 0.05, 0.25, 1 mg

Indications & dosages
➤ *Parkinson's disease*—**Adult:** 0.05 mg PO daily for 1st 2 d; then increase to 0.1-0.15 mg q 3rd d over 12 d. Then increase 0.25 mg q 3rd d prn until optimum response is achieved. Give in divided doses tid.

perphenazine
Apo-Perphenazine*, PMS Perphenazine*, Trilafon, Trilafon Concentrate

Phenothiazine (piperazine derivative); antipsychotic, antiemetic
PRC: C

Available forms
Injection: 5 mg/ml; *Oral concentration:* 16 mg/5 ml; *Syrup:* 2 mg/5 ml*; *Tablets:* 2, 4, 8, 16 mg

Indications & dosages
➤ *Psychosis in nonhospitalized patient*—**Adult:** 4-8 mg PO tid; reduce ASAP to lowest effective dose. **Child > 12 yr:** Lowest adult dose.
➤ *Psychosis in hospitalized patient*—**Adult:** 8-16 mg PO bid-qid; increase to 64 mg/d prn. Or, 5-10 mg IM q 6 hr prn.

Max 30 mg. **Child > 12 yr:** Lowest adult dose.
➤ *Nausea, vomiting*—**Adult:** 8-16 mg PO daily in divided doses to max 24 mg. Or, 5-10 mg IM prn. May give IV; dilute to 0.5 mg/ml with NSS. Max 5 mg.

phenazopyridine hydrochloride (phenylazo diamino pyridine hydrochloride)
Azo-Standard, Baridium, Geridium, Phenazo*, Prodium, Pyridiate, Pyridium, Pyridium Plus, Urodine, Urogesic

Azo dye; urinary tract analgesic
PRC: B

Available forms
Tablets: 95, 100, 150, 200 mg

Indications & dosages
➤ *Pain with urinary tract irritation or UTI*—**Adult:** 200 mg PO tid pc × 2 d. **Child:** 12 mg/kg PO daily in 3 equal doses pc × 2 d.

phenobarbital
Ancalixir*, Barbita, Solfoton

phenobarbital sodium
Luminal Sodium

Barbiturate; anticonvulsant, sedative-hypnotic
PRC: D; CSS: IV

Available forms
Capsules: 16 mg; *Elixir:* 15, 20 mg/5 ml; *Injection:* 30, 60, 65, 130 mg/ml; *Tablets:* 15, 16, 30, 60, 100 mg

Indications & dosages
➤ *Epilepsy, febrile seizures*—**Adult:** 60-200 mg PO daily in divided doses tid or in 1 dose hs. **Child:** 3-6 mg/kg PO daily divided q 12 hr.
➤ *Status epilepticus*—**Adult:** 200-600 mg IV. **Child:** 100-400 mg IV.
➤ *Sedation*—**Adult:** 30-120 mg PO daily in 2-3 divided doses. **Child:** 3-5 mg/kg PO daily in divided doses tid.
➤ *Preop sedation*—**Adult:** 100-200 mg IM 60-90 min preop. **Child:** 16-100 mg IM or 1-3 mg/kg IV, IM, or PO 60-90 min preop.

phenylephrine hydrochloride (systemic)
Neo-Synephrine

Adrenergic; vasoconstrictor
PRC: C

Available forms
Injection: 10 mg/ml

Indications & dosages
➤ *Hypotension*—**Adult:** 2-5 mg SC or IM; repeat in 1-2 hr prn. Or, 0.1-0.5 mg slow IV; repeat in 10-15 min. **Child:** 0.1 mg/kg IM or SC; repeat in 1-2 hr prn.
➤ *Severe hypotension and shock*—**Adult:** 10 mg in 250-500 ml D_5W or NSS. Start infusion at 100-180 mcg/min; decrease to 40-60 mcg/min when BP is stable.

---

phenytoin (diphenylhydantoin)
Dilantin-125, Dilantin Infatabs

phenytoin sodium
Dilantin

phenytoin sodium (extended)
Dilantin Kapseals, Phenytek

Hydantoin derivative; anticonvulsant
PRC: NR

Available forms
phenytoin *Oral suspension:* 125 mg/5 ml; *Tablets (chewable):* 50 mg; **sodium** *Capsules:* 100 mg (92-mg base); *Injection:* 50 mg/ml (46-mg base); **sodium (extended)** *Capsules:* 30 mg (27.6-mg base), 100 mg (92-mg base), 200 mg (184-mg base), 300 mg (276-mg base)

Indications & dosages
➤ *Seizures*—**Adult:** 100 mg PO tid, increase 100 mg PO q 2-4 wk prn. **Child:** 5 mg/kg or 250 mg/m² PO divided bid or tid. Max 300 mg/d.
➤ *Loading dose*—**Adult:** 1 g PO divided into 3 doses given at 2-hr intervals. Or, 10-15 mg/kg IV at rate not > 50 mg/min. **Child:** 5 mg/kg/d PO in 2 or 3 equally divided doses with later dose individualized to max 300 mg/d.
➤ *Status epilepticus*—**Adult:** Loading dose 10-15 mg/kg IV at rate not > 50 mg/min; then maintenance 100 mg PO or IV q 6-8 hr. **Child:** Loading dose 15-20 mg/kg IV at rate ≤ 1-3 mg/kg/min; then individualize maintenance doses.

phytonadione (vitamin K₁)
Mephyton

Vitamin K; blood coagulation modifier
PRC: C

Available forms
Injection (aqueous colloidal solution): 2, 10 mg/ml; *Injection (aqueous dispersion):* 2, 10 mg/ml; *Tablets:* 5 mg

Indications & dosages
➤ *Hypoprothrombinemia from vitamin K malabsorption, drug treatment, excessive vitamin A dose*—**Adult:** 2.5-10 mg PO, SC, or IM; repeat and increase up to 50 mg. **Infant:** 2 mg PO, IM, or SC. **Child:** 5-10 mg PO, IM, or SC.
➤ *Hypoprothrombinemia secondary to oral anticoagulants*—**Adult:** 2.5-10 mg PO, SC, or IM. In emergency, 10-50 mg slow IV at a rate not > 1 mg/min; repeat q 4 hr prn.

pilocarpine hydrochloride
Adsorbocarpine, Isopto Carpine, Miocarpine*, Pilocar

pilocarpine nitrate
Pilagan, P.V. Carpine Liquifilm

Cholinergic agonist; miotic
PRC: C

Available forms
hydrochloride *Ophthalmic gel:* 4%; *Ophthalmic solution:* 0.25, 0.5, 1, 2, 3, 4, 5, 6, 8, 10%; **nitrate** *Ophthalmic solution:* 1, 2, 4%

---

§ Adjust in immunocompromised patients ¶ Adjust in debilitated patients

Indications & dosages
➤ *Open-angle glaucoma*—**Adult, child:** 1 or 2 gtt up to qid, or 1-cm ribbon of 4% gel q hs.
➤ *Acute angle-closure glaucoma*—**Adult, child:** 1 gtt 2% solution q 5-10 min × 3-6 doses; then 1 gtt q 1-3 hr until pressure controlled.
➤ *Mydriasis*—**Adult, child:** 1 gtt 1% solution.

pimecrolimus
Elidel

Topical immunomodulator; topical skin product
PRC: C

Available forms
Cream: 1% in 15-, 30-, and 100-g tubes

Indications & dosages
➤ *Mild to moderate atopic dermatitis in non-immunocompromised patients, in whom conventional therapies are inadequate or contraindicated*—**Adult, child ≥ 2 yr:** Thin layer on affected skin bid; rub in gently and completely.

pioglitazone hydrochloride
Actos

Thiazolidinedione; antidiabetic
PRC: C

Available forms
Tablets: 15, 30, 45 mg

Indications & dosages
➤ *Type 2 DM*—**Adult:** 15 or 30 mg PO daily. Increase dose prn; max 45 mg/d. In combination treatment, max 30 mg/d.

piperacillin sodium
Pipracil

Extended-spectrum PCN, acylamino PCN; antibiotic
PRC: B

Available forms
Injection: 2, 3, 4 g

Indications & dosages
➤ *Systemic infection*—**Adult, child > 12 yr:** 100-300 mg/kg IV or IM daily in divided doses q 4-6 hr. Max 24 g/d.†
➤ *Surgery prophylaxis*—**Adult:** 2 g IV 30-60 min preop.

piperacillin sodium and tazobactam sodium
Zosyn

Extended-spectrum PCN, beta-lactamase inhibitor; antibiotic
PRC: B

Available forms
Powder for injection: 2, 3, 4 g piperacillin and 0.25, 0.375, 0.5 g tazobactam/vial, respectively

Indications & dosages
➤ *Appendicitis; peritonitis; skin, skin-structure infection; postpartum endo-*

metritis; PID; community-acquired pneumonia—**Adult:** 3 g piperacillin and 0.375 g
tazobactam IV q 6 hr × 7-10 d.†
➤ *Nosocomial pneumonia*—**Adult:** 4 g
piperacillin and 0.5 g tazobactam IV q 6 hr
given with an aminoglycoside.†

potassium chloride
K+10, Kaochlor 10%, K-Dur, Klor-Con,
K-Lyte Cl, K-Tab, Slow-K, Ten-K

*Potassium (K+) supplement; therapeutic
agent for electrolyte balance*
PRC: C

Available forms
Capsules (controlled-release): 8, 10 mEq;
Injection concentration: 1.5, 2 mEq/ml;
Injection for IV infusion: 0.1, 0.2, 0.3,
0.4 mEq/ml; *PO liquid:* 20, 30, 40 mEq/
15 ml; *Powder for PO use:* 15, 20, 25 mEq/
packet; *Tablets (controlled-release):* 6.7, 8,
10, 20 mEq; *Tablets (extended-release):* 8,
10 mEq

Indications & dosages
➤ *Prevention of hypokalemia*—**Adult,
child:** 16-24 mEq PO daily divided; adjust
prn.
➤ *Hypokalemia*—**Adult, child:** 40-
100 mEq PO daily in divided bid-qid. Use
IV form when PO is not feasible. Max IV
dose 20 mEq/hr (concentration of
40 mEq/L). Max 150 mEq PO daily for
adult, 3 mEq/kg PO daily for child.
➤ *Severe hypokalemia*—**Adult, child:**
Concentration should be < 80 mEq/L and
given at ≤ 40 mEq/hr IV. Max 150 mEq

IV daily for adult; 3 mEq/kg IV daily or
40 mEq/m² for child.

potassium gluconate
Kaon, Kaylixir, K-G Elixir

*Potassium (K+) supplement; therapeutic
agent for electrolyte balance*
PRC: C

Available forms
Liq: 20 mEq/15 ml; *Tablets:* 500, 595 mg
(83.45 mg and 99 mg potassium, respectively)

Indications & dosages
➤ *Hypokalemia*—**Adult:** 40-100 mEq PO
daily divided bid-qid; 20 mEq daily for
prevention. Adjust prn.

pramipexole
dihydrochloride
Mirapex

*Nonergot dopamine agonist; antiparkin-
sonian*
PRC: C

Available forms
Tablets: 0.125, 0.25, 1, 1.5 mg

Indications & dosages
➤ *Parkinson's disease*—**Adult:** 0.375 mg
PO daily in divided doses tid; increase q
5-7 d. Maintenance 1.5-4.5 mg/d in 3 divided doses.†

---

§ Adjust in immunocompromised patients   ¶ Adjust in debilitated patients

pravastatin sodium (eptastatin)
Pravachol

HMG-CoA reductase inhibitor; anti-lipemic
PRC: X

Available forms
Tablets: 10, 20, 40, 80 mg

Indications & dosages
➤ *Prevention of coronary events; hyperlipidemia*—**Adult:** 40 mg PO daily at same time each d. Adjust dosage q 4 wks prn; max 80 mg/d.†, ‡, §
➤ *Heterozygous familial hypercholesterolemia*—**Child 14-18 yr:** 40 mg PO daily. **Child 8-13 yr:** 20 mg PO daily.†,‡,§

prazosin hydrochloride
Minipress

Alpha blocker; antihypertensive
PRC: C

Available forms
Capsules: 1, 2, 5 mg

Indications & dosages
➤ *HTN*—**Adult:** PO test dose 1 mg hs. Then 1 mg PO bid or tid. Increase slowly. Max 20 mg/d. Maintenance 6-15 mg/d divided tid.

prednisolone
Delta-Cortef, Prelone

prednisolone acetate
Cotolone, Key-Pred 25, Predalone 50, Predcor-50

prednisolone sodium phosphate
Hydeltrasol, Key-Pred SP, Orapred, Pediapred

prednisolone tebutate
Nor-Pred TBA, Predate TBA, Predcor-TBA, Prednisol TBA

Glucocorticoid; anti-inflammatory, immunosuppressant
PRC: C

Available forms
prednisolone *Syrup:* 5, 15 mg/5 ml; *Tablets:* 5 mg; **acetate** *Injection:* 25, 50 mg/ml; **sodium phosphate** *Injection:* 20 mg/ml; *Oral solution:* 5, 15 mg/5 ml; **tebutate** *Injection (suspension):* 20 mg/ml

Indications & dosages
➤ *Severe inflammation, modification of body's immune response to disease*—**prednisolone. Adult:** 2.5-15 mg PO bid-qid. **Child:** 0.14-2 mg/kg/d PO or 4-60 mg/m²/d in 4 divided doses. **prednisolone acetate. Adult:** 2-30 mg IM q 12 hr. **Child:** 0.04-0.25 mg/kg or 1.5-7.5 mg/m² IM daily or bid. **prednisolone sodium phosphate. Adult:** 5-60 mg IM, IV, or PO daily. **Child:** 0.14-2 mg/kg/d or 4-60 mg/m²/d in 3 or 4 divided doses IM, IV, or PO. **pred-

nisolone tebutate. **Adult:** 4-40 mg into joints and lesions prn.

➤ *Acute exacerbations of MS*—**Adult: prednisolone sodium phosphate** 200 mg/d PO × 1 wk, followed by 80 mg q other d.

➤ *Nephrotic syndrome*—**Child: prednisolone sodium phosphate** 60 mg/m²/d PO in 3 divided doses for 4 wk, followed by 4 wk of single-dose alternate-day therapy at 40 mg/m²/d.

➤ *Uncontrolled asthma in patients taking inhaled corticosteroids and long-acting bronchodilators*—**Child: prednisolone sodium phosphate** 1-2 mg/kg/d PO in single or divided doses. Continue short course, or "burst," therapy, until child achieves peak expiratory flow rate of 80% of his or her personal best or symptoms resolve, usually 3-10 d of treatment.

---

prednisone
Liquid Pred, Meticorten, Panasol-S, Prednicen-M, Prednisone Intensol

Adrenocorticoid; anti-inflammatory, immunosuppressant
PRC: C

Available forms
Oral solution: 5 mg/5 ml, 5 mg/ml (concentrate); *Syrup:* 5 mg/5 ml; *Tablets:* 1, 2.5, 5, 10, 20, 50 mg

Indications & dosages
➤ *Inflammation, immunosuppression*—**Adult:** 5-60 mg PO daily in 2-4 divided doses. Maintenance dose daily or q other d. **Child:** 0.14-2 mg/kg or 4-60 mg/m² PO daily in 4 divided doses.

---

primidone
Apo-Primidone*, Mysoline, PMS Primidone*, Sertan*

Barbiturate analogue; anticonvulsant
PRC: NR

Available forms
Oral suspension: 250 mg/5 ml; *Tablets:* 50, 250 mg

Indications & dosages
➤ *Seizures*—**Adult, child ≥ 8 yr:** 100-125 mg PO hs on d 1-3; 100-125 mg PO bid on d 4-6; 100-125 mg PO tid on d 7-9; then 250 mg PO tid. Increase to 250 mg qid prn. Max 2 g/d in divided doses. **Child < 8 yr:** 50 mg PO hs × 3 d; then 50 mg PO bid on d 4-6, 100 mg PO bid on d 7-9; then 125-250 mg PO tid.

---

probenecid
Benemid, Benuryl*

Sulfonamide derivative; uricosuric
PRC: NR

Available forms
Tablets: 500 mg

Indications & dosages
➤ *Gonorrhea*—**Adult:** 3.5 g ampicillin PO with 1 g probenecid PO; or 1 g probenecid PO 30 min before dose of 4.8 million units aqueous PCN G procaine IM; inject at 2 different sites.
➤ *Hyperuricemia of gout, gouty arthritis*—**Adult:** 250 mg PO bid × 1 wk; then 500 mg bid. Max 2 g/d.

---

§ Adjust in immunocompromised patients   ¶ Adjust in debilitated patients

➤ *Prevent RF after cidofovir infusion—*
Adult: 2 g PO 3 hr before cidofovir infusion; then 1 g PO 2 and 8 hr after infusion.

procainamide hydrochloride
Procanbid, Promine, Pronestyl

Procaine derivative; ventricular and supraventricular antiarrhythmic
PRC: C

Available forms
Capsules: 250, 375, 500 mg; *Injection:* 100, 500 mg/ml; *Tablets:* 250, 375, 500 mg; *Tablets (extended-release):* 250, 500, 750, 1,000 mg

Indications & dosages
➤ *Ventricular arrhythmias—***Adult:** 100 mg slow IV push q 5 min until arrhythmias disappear, adverse reactions develop, or 500 mg given. Continue infusion of 2-6 mg/min. If arrhythmias recur, repeat bolus and increase infusion rate. Or, 50 mg/kg IM divided q 3-6 hr; for arrhythmias during surgery, 100-500 mg IM. PO: 50 mg/kg/d in divided doses q 3 hr. May divide extended-release PO forms q 6 or 12 hr based on product.†

prochlorperazine
Compazine, PMS Prochlorperazine*

prochlorperazine edisylate
Compazine, Cotranzine, Ultrazine-10

prochlorperazine maleate
Compazine, PMS Prochlorperazine*, Stemetil*

Phenothiazine (piperazine derivative); antipsychotic, antiemetic, anxiolytic
PRC: NR

Available forms
prochlorperazine *Injection:* 5 mg/ml; *Suppository:* 2.5, 5, 25 mg; *Tablets:* 5, 10 mg; **edisylate** *Injection:* 5 mg/ml; *Syrup:* 5 mg/5 ml; **maleate** *Capsules (extended-release):* 10, 15, 30 mg; *Tablets:* 5, 10, 25 mg

Indications & dosages
➤ *Preop nausea—***Adult:** 5-10 mg IM 1-2 hr before anesthesia; repeat once in 30 min prn. Or, 5-10 mg IV 15-30 min before anesthesia; repeat once prn.
➤ *Nausea, vomiting—***Adult:** 5-10 mg PO tid or qid; 25 mg PR bid; 5-10 mg IM, repeat q 3-4 hr prn. Or, 2.5-10 mg IV at max rate 5 mg/min. **Child 9-13 kg:** 2.5 mg PO or PR daily or bid. Or, 0.132 mg/kg IM. **Child 14-17 kg:** 2.5 mg PO or PR bid or tid. Or, 0.132 mg/kg deep IM. **Child 18-39 kg:** 2.5 mg PO or PR tid; or 5 mg PO or PR bid. Or, 0.132 mg/kg deep IM.
➤ *Psychotic disorders—***Adult:** 5-10 mg PO tid or qid. **Child 2-12 yr:** 2.5 mg PO or PR bid or tid. Max 10 mg on d 1. Increase dose prn. Child 2-10 yr, max 25 mg/d.
➤ *Anxiety—***Adult:** 5-10 mg deep IM q 3-4 hr; max 20 mg/d. Treat ≤ 12 wk. Or, 5-10 mg PO tid-qid. Or, 15 mg extended-release capsules daily or 10 mg extended-release capsules q 12 hr.

---

progesterone
Prometrium

Progestin; hormonal agent
PRC: B

Available forms
Capsules: 100, 200 mg; *Injection (oil):*
50 mg/ml

Indications & dosages
➤ *Prevent endometrial hyperplasia in postmenopausal patient with intact uterus*—**Adult:** 200 mg PO q pm × 12 d in 28 d cycle.
➤ *Amenorrhea*—**Adult:** 400 mg PO q pm × 10 d.

promethazine hydrochloride
Anergan 50, Phenergan

Phenothiazine derivative; antiemetic, antivertigo drug, H₁-receptor antagonist, adjunct to analgesics, sedative
PRC: C

Available forms
Injection: 25, 50 mg/ml; *Suppository:* 12.5, 25, 50 mg; *Syrup:* 6.25 mg/5 ml; *Tablets:* 12.5, 25, 50 mg

Indications & dosages
➤ *Motion sickness*—**Adult:** 25 mg PO bid. **Child:** 12.5-25 mg PO, IM, or PR bid.
➤ *Nausea*—**Adult:** 12.5-25 mg PO, IM, or PR q 4-6 hr prn. **Child:** 12.5-25 mg IM or PR q 4-6 hr prn.
➤ *Rhinitis, allergy symptoms*—**Adult:** 12.5 mg PO qid; or 25 mg PO hs. **Child:**

6.25-12.5 mg PO tid or 25 mg PO or PR hs.
➤ *Sedation*—**Adult:** 25-50 mg PO or IM hs or prn. **Child:** 12.5-25 mg PO, IM, or PR hs.
➤ *Preop or postop sedation, adjunct to analgesics*—**Adult:** 25-50 mg IM, IV, or PO. **Child:** 12.5-25 mg IM, IV, or PO.

propafenone hydrochloride
Rythmol

Sodium channel antagonist; antiarrhythmic
PRC: C

Available forms
Tablets: 150, 225, 300 mg

Indications & dosages
➤ *Ventricular arrhythmias*—**Adult:** 150 mg PO q 8 hr. May increase dose q 3-4 d; max 225 mg q 8 hr. If needed, 300 mg q 8 hr. Max 900 mg/d.

propofol
Diprivan

Phenol derivative; anesthetic
PRC: B

Available forms
Injection: 10 mg/ml in 20-ml amp; 50-ml prefilled syringes; 50-, 100-ml infusion vials

Indications & dosages
➤ *Sedation in mechanically ventilated patient*—**Adult:** 5 mcg/kg/min × 5 min. Increase rate q 5-10 min in 5-10 mcg/kg/

min increments prn. Rates of 5-50 mcg/
kg/min or more may be needed.

propoxyphene hydrochloride
Darvon, 692*, Darvon Pulvules

propoxyphene napsylate
Darvon-N

Opioid analgesic; opioid analgesic
PRC: C; CSS IV

Available forms
hydrochloride *Capsules:* 65 mg; **napsylate** *Oral suspension:* 50 mg/5 ml; *Tablets:* 100 mg

Indications & dosages
➤ *Pain*—**Adult: hydrochloride** 65 mg PO q 4 hr prn. Max 390 mg/d. Or, **napsylate** 100 mg PO q 4 hr prn. Max 600 mg/d.

propranolol hydrochloride
Detensol*, Inderal, Inderal LA,
InnoPran XL, Novopranol*

Beta blocker; antihypertensive, antianginal, antiarrhythmic, adjunctive treatment for MI
PRC: C

Available forms
Capsules (extended-release): 60, 80, 120, 180 mg; *Injection:* 1 mg/ml; *Oral solution:* 4, 8, 80 (concentrate) mg/ml; *Tablets:* 10, 20, 40, 60, 80, 90 mg

Indications & dosages
➤ *Angina*—**Adult:** Total daily dose 80-320 mg PO bid-qid; or one 80-mg extended-release capsule daily. Increase q 7-10 d.
➤ *MI*—**Adult:** 180-240 mg PO tid or qid 5-21 d post-MI.
➤ *Supraventricular, ventricular arrhythmias; tachyarrhythmias during anesthesia*—**Adult:** 0.5-3 mg slow IV push (≤ 1 mg/min). After 3 mg, next dose in 2 min; additional doses in > 4-hr intervals. Maintenance 10-30 mg PO tid or qid.
➤ *HTN*—**Adult:** 80 mg PO daily in 2-4 divided doses or extended-release (InnoPran XL) q hs. Increase q 3-7 d. Max 640 mg/d. Maintenance 160-480 mg/d.
➤ *Essential tremor*—**Adult:** 40 mg PO bid. Maintenance 120-320 mg/d in 3 divided doses.
➤ *Hypertrophic subaortic stenosis*—**Adult:** 20-40 mg PO tid or qid, or 80-160 mg extended-release capsules in 1 dose/d.
➤ *Pheochromocytoma*—**Adult:** 60 mg PO daily in divided doses with an alpha blocker 3 d preop.

propylthiouracil (PTU)
Propyl-Thyracil*

Thyroid hormone antagonist; antihyperthyroid
PRC: D

Available forms
Tablets: 50 mg

Indications & dosages
➤ *Hyperthyroidism*—**Adult:** 300-450 mg daily in divided doses. Continue until pa-

tient is euthyroid, then, maintenance 100 mg PO once daily divided tid. **Child > 10 yr:** 100 mg PO tid. Continue until patient is euthyroid, then individualize maintenance dose. **Child 6-10 yr:** 50-150 mg PO daily in divided doses q 8 hr. Continue until patient is euthyroid, then individualize maintenance dose. **Neonates:** 5-7 mg/kg daily in divided doses q 8 hr.

➤ *Thyrotoxic crisis*—**Adult:** 200 mg PO q 4-6 hr on d 1. Reduce dose to maintenance level.

protamine sulfate

Antidote; heparin antagonist
PRC: C

Available forms
Injection: 10 mg/ml

Indications & dosages
➤ *Heparin overdose*—**Adult:** Dose based on blood coagulation studies, usually 1 mg for each 90-115 units heparin. Max 50 mg.

pseudoephedrine hydrochloride
Cenafed, Decofed, Dimetapp, Efidac/24, Genaphed, PediaCare Infants' Decongestant, Sudafed, Triaminic

pseudoephedrine sulfate
Drixoral 12 Hour Non-Drowsy Formula

Adrenergic; decongestant
PRC: C

Available forms
Hydrochloride *Capsules:* 60 mg; *Capsules (liquid gel):* 30 mg; *Oral solution:* 7.5 mg/0.8 ml, 15 mg/5 ml, 30 mg/5 ml; *Tablets:* 30, 60 mg; *Tablets (chewable):* 15 mg; *Tablets (controlled-release):* 240 mg; *Tablets (extended-release):* 120, 240 mg; **pseudoephedrine sulfate** *Tablets (extended-release):* 240 mg

Indications & dosages
➤ *Decongestant*—**Adult, adolescent ≥ 12 yr:** 60 mg PO q 4-6 hr; or 120 mg PO extended-release tablet q 12 hr; or 240 mg PO controlled-release tablet daily. Max 240 mg daily. **Child 6-12 yr:** 30 mg PO q 4-6 hr. Max 120 mg daily. **Child 2-5 yr:** 15 mg PO q 4-6 hr. Max 60 mg daily. Or, 4 mg/kg or 125 mg/m² PO divided qid.

pyridoxine hydrochloride (vitamin B₆)
Beesix, Nestrex, Rodex

H₂O-soluble vitamin; nutritional supplement
PRC: A

Available forms
Capsules: 500 mg; *Capsules, tablets (timed-release):* 100 mg; *Injection:* 100 mg/ml; *Tablets:* 10, 25, 50, 100, 200, 250, 500 mg

Indications & dosages
➤ *Dietary vitamin B₆ deficiency*—**Adult:** 10-20 mg PO, IM, or IV daily × 3 wk; then 2-5 mg/d as supplement to proper diet.

➤ *Seizures related to vitamin B₆ deficiency or dependency*—**Adult, child:** 100 mg IM or IV in 1 dose.

➤ *Prevent isoniazid pyridoxine deficiency*—**Adult:** 10-50 mg PO daily.

➤ *Isoniazid toxicity (> 10 g)*—**Adult:** Give equal amounts pyridoxine: Generally 1-4 g IV, then 1 g IM q 30 min until entire dose is given.

quetiapine fumarate
Seroquel

Dibenzapine derivative; antipsychotic
PRC: C

Available forms
Tablets: 25, 100, 200, 300 mg

Indications & dosages
➤ *Psychotic disorders*—**Adult:** 25 mg bid. Increase by 25-50 mg bid or tid on d 2 and 3, as tolerated. Target dose 300-400 mg daily, divided bid or tid, by d 4. Adjust dose q ≥ 2 d prn. **Elderly:** Lower doses, slow adjustment; carefully monitor in initial dose period. Adjust dose in hypotensive patient.†, ¶

quinapril hydrochloride
Accupril

ACE inhibitor; antihypertensive
PRC: C (D, 2nd and 3rd trimesters)

Available forms
Tablets: 5, 10, 20, 40 mg

Indications & dosages
➤ *HTN*—**Adult ≤ 65 yr:** 10 or 20 mg PO daily or 5 mg/d if patient is using diuretic.† **Adult > 65 yr:** Initially 10 mg PO daily; adjust q 2 wk prn.†

➤ *HF*—**Adult:** 5 mg PO bid. Increase at wkly intervals. Max 20 mg bid.†

quinidine gluconate
Quinaglute Dura-Tabs, Quinalan, Quinate*

quinidine sulfate
Apo-Quinidine*, Cin-Quin, Quinidex Extentabs

Cinchona alkaloid; anti-tachyarrhythmic
PRC: C

Available forms
gluconate *Injection:* 80 mg/ml; *Tablets (extended-release):* 324, 325*, 330 mg; **sulfate** *Injection:* 200 mg/ml*; *Tablets, capsules:* 200, 300 mg; *Tablets (extended-release):* 300 mg

Indications & dosages
➤ *Atrial fibrillation, flutter*—**Adult:** 200 mg PO q 2-3 hr × 5-8 doses; then increase daily. Max 3-4 g/d.

➤ *PSVT*—**Adult:** 400-600 mg IM or PO q 2-3 hr.

➤ *PAC; PVC; PAT; PVT; maintenance after cardioversion of atrial fibrillation*—**Adult:** Test dose 200 mg PO or IM; then 200-400 mg (sulfate or equivalent base) PO q 4-6 hr. Or, 600 mg (gluconate) IM; then 400 mg q 2 hr prn. Or, 800 mg (gluconate) in 40 ml D₅W IV at 16 mg/min. **Child:** Test dose 2 mg/kg PO; then 30 mg/

kg/24 hr PO or 900 mg/m²/24 hr PO in 5 divided doses.

quinupristin and dalfopristin
Synercid

Streptogramin; antibiotic
PRC: B

Available forms
Injection: 500 mg/10 ml (150 mg quinupristin, 350 mg dalfopristin)

Indications & dosages
➤ *Vancomycin-resistant* Enterococcus faecium *bacteremia*—**Adult, adolescent ≥ 16 yr:** 7.5 mg/kg IV over 1 hr q 8 hr.
➤ *Skin, skin-structure infection from* Staphylococcus aureus *(methicillin susceptible) or* Streptococcus pyogenes—**Adult, adolescent ≥ 16 yr:** 7.5 mg/kg IV over 1 hr q 12 hr ≥ 7 d.

rabeprazole sodium
Aciphex

Proton pump inhibitor; antiulcerative
PRC: B

Available forms
Tablets (delayed-release): 20 mg

Indications & dosages
➤ *GERD*—**Adult:** 20 mg PO daily × 4-8 wk. May continue another 8 wk prn.
➤ *Maintain healing of GERD*—**Adult:** 20 mg PO daily.
➤ *Duodenal ulcers*—**Adult:** 20 mg PO daily in am pc ≤ 4 wk.

➤ *Hypersecretory conditions (Zollinger-Ellison syndrome)*—**Adult:** 60 mg PO daily; increase prn to 100 PO daily or 60 mg PO bid.
➤ *Symptomatic GERD, including daytime and nighttime heartburn*—**Adult:** 20 mg PO daily × 4 wk. May continue another 4 wk prn.
➤ *Prevent recurrence due to* Helicobacter pylori *infection*—20 mg PO bid with amoxicillin 1,000 mg PO bid and clarithromycin 500 mg PO bid × 7 d.

raloxifene hydrochloride
Evista

Selective estrogen receptor modulator; antiosteoporotic
PRC: X

Available forms
Tablets: 60 mg

Indications & dosages
➤ *Prevent osteoporosis*—**Adult:** 60 mg PO daily.

ramipril
Altace

ACE inhibitor; antihypertensive
PRC: C (D, 2nd and 3rd trimesters)

Available forms
Capsules: 1.25, 2.5, 5, 10 mg

Indications & dosages
➤ *HTN*—**Adult:** 2.5 mg PO daily for patient not using diuretic; 1.25 mg PO daily

---

§ Adjust in immunocompromised patients   ¶ Adjust in debilitated patients

for patient using diuretic. Increase prn. Maintenance 2.5-20 mg/d in single dose or divided bid.†

➤ *HF*—**Adult:** 2.5 mg PO bid. If hypotension, decrease to 1.25 mg PO bid. May increase to max 5 mg PO bid prn.†

➤ *Reduce risk of MI, stroke, death from CV causes*—**Adult ≥ 55 yr:** 2.5 mg PO daily × 1 wk, then 5 mg PO daily × 3 wk. Increase to maintenance dose of 10 mg PO daily. For HTN or recent MI patient, divide daily dose.†

ranitidine hydrochloride
Apo-Ranitidine*, Zantac, Zantac-C*, Zantac EFFERdose, Zantac 75

H_2-receptor antagonist; antiulcerative
PRC: B

Available forms
Capsules: 150, 300 mg; *Injection:* 1 mg/ml premixed in 50 ml of ½ NSS, 25 mg/ml in 2- and 6-ml vials; *Syrup:* 15 mg/ml; *Tablets:* 75, 150, 300 mg; *Tablets/granules (effervescent):* 150 mg

Indications & dosages
➤ *Duodenal, gastric ulcer; hypersecretory conditions (Zollinger-Ellison syndrome)*—**Adult:** 150 mg PO bid or 300 mg/d hs. Or, 50 mg IV or IM q 6-8 hr. For Zollinger-Ellison syndrome, max 6 g PO daily.†

➤ *Maintenance treatment for duodenal, gastric ulcer*—**Adult:** 150 mg PO hs.†

➤ *GERD*—**Adult:** 150 mg PO bid.†

repaglinide
Prandin

Meglitinide; antidiabetic
PRC: C

Available forms
Tablets: 0.5, 1, 2 mg

Indications & dosages
➤ *Type 2 DM, alone or with metformin, rosiglitazone maleate, or pioglitazone HCl*—**Adult patient not previously treated or with HbA_{1c} < 8%:** 0.5 mg PO up to 30 min each ac.† **Adult patient previously on glucose-lowering drugs and HbA_{1c} ≥ 8%:** 1-2 mg PO up to 30 min each ac. Range 0.5-4 mg with meals divided bid-qid. Max 16 mg/d.†

riboflavin (vitamin B₂)

H_2O-soluble vitamin; vitamin B complex vitamin
PRC: NR

Available forms
Tablets: 25, 50, 100 mg; *Tablets (sugar-free):* 50, 100 mg

Indications & dosages
➤ *Riboflavin deficiency; polyneuritis, cheilosis secondary to pellagra*—**Adult, child ≥ 12 yr:** 5-30 mg PO daily. **Child < 12 yr:** 3-10 mg PO daily.

---

rifabutin
Mycobutin

Semisynthetic ansamycin; antibiotic
PRC: B

Available forms
Capsules: 150 mg

Indications & dosages
➤ *Prevent disseminated MAC in HIV infection*—**Adult:** 300 mg PO daily in 1 dose or divided bid with food.

rifampin
Rifadin, Rifadin IV, Rimactane, Rofact*

Semisynthetic rifamycin B derivative (macrocyclic antibiotic); antituberculotic
PRC: C

Available forms
Capsules: 150, 300 mg; *Injection:* 600 mg

Indications & dosages
➤ *Pulmonary TB*—**Adult:** 600 mg/d PO or IV 1 hr ac or 2 hr pc. **Child > 5 yr:** 10-20 mg/kg PO or IV daily 1 hr ac or 2 hr pc. Max 600 mg/d.
➤ *Meningococcal carriers*—**Adult:** 600 mg PO or IV bid × 2 d, or 600 mg/d PO or IV daily × 4 d. **Child 1 mo-12 yr:** 10 mg/kg PO or IV bid × 2 d, ≤ 600 mg/d, or 10-20 mg/kg/d × 4 d. **Neonate:** 5 mg/kg PO or IV bid × 2 d.
➤ *Haemophilus influenzae type b prophylaxis*—**Adult, child:** 20 mg/kg/d PO × 4 d; max 600 mg/d.

rifapentine
Priftin

RNA polymerase inhibitor; antituberculotic
PRC: C

Available forms
Tablets (film-coated): 150 mg

Indications & dosages
➤ *Pulmonary TB*—**Adult:** Intensive phase, 600 mg PO 2 times/wk × 2 mo, doses ≥ 72 hr apart. For continuation phase, 600 mg PO q wk × 4 mo.

risedronate sodium
Actonel

Bisphosphonate; antiresorptive drug
PRC: C

Available forms
Tablets: 5, 30, 35 mg

Indications & dosages
➤ *Prevent and treat postmenopausal osteoporosis*—**Adult:** 5 mg PO daily or 35-mg tablet q wk ≥ 30 min before 1st food or liq of d. Take while upright with 6-8 oz water.
➤ *Prevent and treat glucocorticoid-induced osteoporosis*—**Adult:** 5 mg PO daily ≥ 30 min before 1st food or liq of d. Take while upright with 6-8 oz water.
➤ *Paget's disease*—**Adult:** 30 mg PO daily × 2 mo. If treatment fails, may repeat ≥ 2 mo after completing 1st treatment.

§ Adjust in immunocompromised patients ¶ Adjust in debilitated patients

risperidone
Risperdal, Risperdal M-Tab

Benzisoxazole derivative; antipsychotic
PRC: C

Available forms
Oral solution: 1 mg/ml; *Tablets:* 0.25, 0.5, 1, 2, 3, 4 mg; *Tablets (orally disintegrating):* 0.5, 1, 2 mg

Indications & dosages
➤ *Short-term (6-8 wk) treatment of schizophrenia*—**Adult:** 1 mg PO bid. Increase by 1 mg bid on d 2 and 3 to target dose of 3 mg bid. Or, 1 mg PO on d 1; 2 mg PO on d 2; and 4 mg PO on d 3. Wait at least 1 wk before adjusting dosage further. Adjust doses by 1-2 mg up to 8 mg/d.†,‡,¶
➤ *Delay relapse in long-term (1-2 yr) treatment of schizophrenia*—**Adult:** 1 mg PO on d 1; 2 mg on d 2; and 4 mg on d 3. Range 2-8 mg daily.†,‡,¶
Note: **Elderly or patients at risk of hypotension:** Give 0.5 mg PO bid. Increase by 0.5 mg bid. Give increases > 1.5 mg bid at intervals of at least 1 wk. Subsequent switches to daily dosing may be made after patient is using bid regimen for 2-3 days at target dose.

ritonavir
Norvir

HIV protease inhibitor; antiviral
PRC: B

Available forms
Capsules: 100 mg; *Oral solution:* 80 mg/ml

Indications & dosages
➤ *HIV infection*—**Adult:** 600 mg PO bid ac. If patient is nauseous, give 300 mg bid × 1 d, 400 mg bid × 2 d, 500 mg bid × 1 d, and 600 mg bid thereafter.

rivastigmine tartrate
Exelon

Cholinesterase inhibitor; cholinomimetic
PRC: B

Available forms
Capsules: 1.5, 3, 4.5, 6 mg; *Solution:* 2 mg/ml

Indications & dosages
➤ *Alzheimer's disease*—**Adult:** 1.5 mg PO bid with food. Increase to 3 mg bid after 2 wk, as tolerated; then increase to 4.5 mg bid and 6 mg bid as tolerated after 2 wk on previous dose. Range 6-12 mg/d; max 12 mg/d.

rofecoxib
Vioxx

Cyclooxygenase-2 inhibitor; nonopioid analgesic, anti-inflammatory
PRC: C

Available forms
Oral suspension: 12.5 mg/5 ml, 25 mg/5 ml; *Tablets:* 12.5, 25, 50 mg

Indications & dosages
➤ *OA*—**Adult:** 12.5 mg PO daily, increase prn to max 25 mg PO daily.
➤ *Pain, treatment of primary dysmenorrhea*—**Adult:** 50 mg PO daily prn ≤ 5 d.

➤ *RA*—**Adult:** 25 mg PO daily. Max
25 mg/d.

ropinirole hydrochloride
Requip

*Nonergoline dopamine agonist; anti-
parkinsonian*
PRC: C

Available forms
Tablets: 0.25, 0.5, 1, 2, 5 mg

Indications & dosages
➤ *Parkinson's disease*—**Adult:** 0.25 mg
PO tid. Adjust wkly. After wk 4, may increase by 1.5 mg/d wkly up to 9 mg/d;
then increase wkly up to 3 mg/d. Max
24 mg/d.

rosiglitazone maleate
Avandia

Thiazolidinedione; antidiabetic
PRC: C

Available forms
Tablets: 2, 4, 8 mg

Indications & dosages
➤ *Type 2 DM alone, or with metformin,
or with sulfonylureas*—**Adult:** 4 mg PO
daily in am or in divided doses bid in am
and pm. May increase to 8 mg PO daily or
in divided doses bid after 12 wk of treatment.

rosiglitazone maleate and
metformin hydrochloride
Avandamet

Thiazolidinedione/biguanide; antidiabetic
PRC: C

Available forms
Tablets: 1, 2, 4 mg rosiglitazone maleate/
500 mg metformin hydrochloride

Indications & dosages
➤ *Type 2 DM inadequately controlled on
metformin and/or rosiglitazone*—**Adult:**
Dose individualized bid with meals based
on patient's current doses of rosiglitazone
or metformin. If using metformin alone,
2 mg rosiglitazone PO bid, plus dose of
metformin already being taken (500 or
1,000 mg PO bid). May increase dose after
8-12 wk. If using rosiglitazone alone,
500 mg metformin PO bid, plus dose of
rosiglitazone already being taken (2 or 4 mg
PO bid). May increase dose after 1-2 wk.
Note: Total daily dose of Avandamet may
be increased in increments of 4 mg rosiglitazone or 500 mg metformin, or both, up
to max daily dose 8 mg/2,000 mg in 2 divided doses. **Elderly:** Initial and maintenance doses should be conservative.

salmeterol xinafoate
Serevent Diskus

*Selective beta$_2$-adrenergic agonist; bron-
chodilator*
PRC: C

Available forms
Inhalation powder: 50 mcg/blister

---

§ Adjust in immunocompromised patients ¶ Adjust in debilitated patients

Indications & dosages

➤ *Asthma, prevent bronchospasm for nocturnal asthma or reversible obstructive airway disease*—**Adult, child ≥ 4 yr:** 1 inhalation in am and pm, approximately 12 hr apart.

➤ *COPD, emphysema*—**Adult:** 1 inhalation in am and pm, approximately 12 hr apart.

---

saquinavir
Fortovase

saquinavir mesylate
Invirase

Protease inhibitor; antiviral
PRC: B

Available forms
saquinavir *Capsules (soft gelatin):* 200 mg; **mesylate** *Capsules (hard gelatin):* 200 mg

Indications & dosages
➤ *HIV infection*—**Adult:** 600 mg (Invirase) or 1,200 mg (Fortovase) PO tid within 2 hr pc.

---

sargramostim (granulocyte macrophage-colony stimulating factor, GM-CSF)
Leukine, Leukine Liquid

Biological response modifier; colony-stimulating factor
PRC: C

Available forms
Injection: 500 mcg/ml; *Powder for injection:* 250 mcg

Indications & dosages
➤ *Acceleration of hematopoiesis after autologous bone marrow transplant (BMT)*—**Adult:** 250 mcg/m^2/d IV over 2 hr × 21 d starting 2-4 hr after BMT.

➤ *BMT failure, engraftment delay*—**Adult:** 250 mcg/m^2/d IV over 2 hr × 14 d. May repeat dose after 7 d of no treatment.

---

scopolamine (hyoscine)
Isopto Hyoscine, Transderm-Scop

scopolamine butylbromide (hyoscine butylbromide)
Buscopan*

scopolamine hydrobromide (hyoscine hydrobromide)

Anticholinergic; antimuscarinic, cycloplegic mydriatic
PRC: C

Available forms
scopolamine *Transdermal patch:* 1.5 mg/2.5 cm^2 (1 mg/72 hr); **butylbromide** *Capsules:* 0.25 mg; *Suppository, tablets*:* 10 mg; **hydrobromide** *Injection:* 0.3, 0.4, 0.5, 0.6, 1 mg/ml in 1-ml vials and ampules, 0.86 mg/ml in 0.5-ml ampules

Indications & dosages
➤ *Spastic states*—**Adult:** 10-20 mg PO tid or qid. Adjust dose prn. Or, 10-20 mg (**butylbromide**) SC, IM, or IV tid or qid.

---

*Canadian   † Adjust in renal impairment   ‡ Adjust in liver impairment

➤ *Delirium, preanesthetic sedation and obstetric amnesia with analgesics*— **Adult:** 0.3-0.65 mg IM, SC, or IV. **Child:** 0.006 mg/kg IM, SC, IV; max 0.3 mg.

➤ *Motion sickness*—**Adult:** 1 Transderm-Scop patch applied to skin behind ear several hr before antiemetic required. Or, **hydrobromide** 300-600 mcg SC, IM, or IV. **Child: hydrobromide** 6 mcg/kg or 200 mcg/m^2 SC, IM, or IV.

selegiline hydrochloride
Atapryl, Carbex, Eldepryl, Selpak

MAO-B inhibitor; antiparkinsonian
PRC: C

Available forms
Capsules: 5 mg; *Tablets:* 5 mg

Indications & dosages
➤ *Parkinson's disease*—**Adult:** 10 mg/d (5 mg at breakfast and 5 mg at lunch). After 2-3 d, slowly decrease levodopa-carbidopa dose.

sertraline hydrochloride
Zoloft

SSRI; antidepressant
PRC: B

Available forms
Oral concentrate: 20 mg/ml; *Tablets:* 25, 50, 100 mg

Indications & dosages
➤ *Depression*—**Adult:** 50 mg/d PO; adjust dose prn at ≥ 1-wk intervals.

➤ *OCD*—**Adult:** 50 mg/d PO. Max 200 mg/d. Adjust dose at ≥ 1-wk intervals.

➤ *Posttraumatic stress disorder, social anxiety disorder*—**Adult:** 25 mg PO daily. Increase to 50 mg PO daily after 1 wk. Adjust dose q wk to max 200 mg/d. Maintain patient on lowest effective dose.‡

➤ *PMDD*—**Adult:** 50 mg PO daily continuously or limited to luteal phase. May increase at 50 mg increments/menstrual cycle up to 150 mg daily for continuous dosing or 100 mg daily for luteal phase dosing. If a 100-mg daily has been established for luteal phase dosing, a 50-mg daily adjustment step for 3 d should be used at the beginning of each luteal phase dosing period.

sibutramine hydrochloride monohydrate
Meridia

SSRI, dopamine and norepinephrine reuptake inhibitor; antiobesity drug
PRC: C; CSS: IV

Available forms
Capsules: 5, 10, 15 mg

Indications & dosages
➤ *Obesity*—**Adult:** 10 mg PO daily. Increase to 15 mg PO daily after 4 wk prn. Reduce to 5 mg PO daily if 10-mg dose not tolerated. Max 15 mg/d.

---

§ Adjust in immunocompromised patients   ¶ Adjust in debilitated patients

sildenafil citrate
Viagra

Selective cyclic guanosine monophos-phate-specific phosphodiesterase type 5 inhibitor; erectile dysfunction treatment
PRC: B

Available forms
Tablets: 25, 50, 100 mg

Indications & dosages
➤ *Erectile dysfunction*—**Adult < 65 yr:** 50 mg PO prn 1 hr before sexual activity. Range 25-100 mg. Max 1 dose daily. **Elderly:** 25 mg PO prn 1 hr before sexual activity. Adjust prn. Max 1 dose daily.†,‡

simvastatin
Zocor

HMG-CoA reductase inhibitor; antilipemic
PRC: X

Available forms
Tablets: 5, 10, 20, 40, 80 mg

Indications & dosages
➤ *Prevent CAD; hyperlipidemia*—**Adult:** 20-40 mg PO daily in pm. Adjust dose at intervals ≥ 4 wk prn; dose range 5-80 mg/d.†
➤ *Homozygous familial hypercholesterol-emia*—**Adult:** 40 mg PO daily in pm or 80 mg PO daily in 3 divided doses (20, 20, and 40 mg in pm).† **Patient using cyclo-sporine:** 5 mg PO daily; max 10 mg/d. **Patient using fibrates or niacin:** max 10 mg PO daily. **Patient using amiodarone or verapamil:** Max 20 mg PO daily.

➤ *Heterozygous familial hypercholester-olemia*—**Child 10-17 yr:** 10 mg PO q pm. Max 40 mg/d.

sodium bicarbonate
Bell/ans, Citrocarbonate, Soda Mint

Alkalinizer; systemic and urinary alkalinizer
PRC: C

Available forms
Tablets: 325, 650 mg; *Injection:* 4% (2.4 mEq/5 ml), 4.2% (5 mEq/10 ml), 5% (297.5 mEq/500 ml), 7.5% (8.92 mEq/ 10 ml and 44.6 mEq/50 ml), 8.4% (10 mEq/10 ml and 50 mEq/50 ml)

Indications & dosages
➤ *Cardiac arrest*—**Adult:** Not routinely recommended; 300-500 ml 5% solution or 200-300 mEq 7.5% or 8.4% solution rapid IV. Base further doses on subsequent blood gas values. Or, 1 mEq/kg dose; repeat 0.5 mEq/kg q 10 min. **Child ≤ 2 yr:** 1 mEq/kg IV or intraosseous injection of 4.2%-8.4% solution. Administer slowly. Max 8 mEq/kg/d.
➤ *Severe metabolic acidosis*—**Adult:** Dose depends on CO_2, pH, and clinical condition. Generally, 90-180 mEq/L IV during 1st hr; adjust prn.
➤ *Metabolic acidosis*—**Adult, child ≥ 12 yr:** 2-5 mEq/kg as 4-8 hr IV infusion.
➤ *Urinary alkalization*—**Adult:** 48 mEq (4 g) PO, then 12-24 mEq (1-2 g) q 4 hr. May need doses of 30-48 mEq (2.5-4 g) q 4 hr, up to 192 mEq (16 g)/d. **Child:** 1-10 mEq (84-840 mg)/kg daily PO.
➤ *Antacid*—**Adult:** 300 mg-2 g PO daily-qid.

---

sodium polystyrene sulfonate
Kayexalate, SPS

Cation-exchange resin; potassium-removing resin
PRC: C

Available forms
Powder: 1-pound jar (3.5 g/tsp); *Suspension:* 15 g/60 ml

Indications & dosages
➤ *Hyperkalemia*—**Adult:** 15 g PO daily-qid in H_2O or sorbitol (3-4 ml/g resin). Or, mix powder and instill through NG tube. Or, 30-50 g/100 ml sorbitol q 6 hr as warm emulsion 20 cm into sigmoid colon. **Child:** 1 g/kg body wt/dose PO or PR prn. PO route preferred.

sotalol
Betapace, Betapace AF, Sotacor*

Beta blocker; antiarrhythmic
PRC: B

Available forms
Tablets: 80, 120, 160, 240 mg

Indications & dosages
➤ *Ventricular arrhythmias*—**Adult:** 80 mg PO bid. Increase q 2-3 d prn; range 160-320 mg/d.†
➤ *Maintain normal sinus rhythm in symptomatic atrial fibrillation or flutter*—**Adult:** 80 mg PO bid (Betapace AF only). Increase prn to 120 mg PO bid after 3 d if QTc interval is < 500 milliseconds. Max 160 mg PO bid.†

spironolactone
Aldactone, Novo-Spiroton*

Potassium-sparing diuretic; antihypertensive, diuretic
PRC: NR

Available forms
Tablets: 25, 50, 100 mg

Indications & dosages
➤ *Edema*—**Adult:** 25-200 mg PO daily or in divided doses. **Child:** 3.3 mg/kg PO daily or in divided doses.
➤ *HTN*—**Adult:** 50-100 mg PO daily or in divided doses.
➤ *Diuretic-induced hypokalemia*—**Adult:** 25-100 mg PO daily.

streptokinase
Streptase

Plasminogen activator; thrombolytic enzyme
PRC: C

Available forms
Injection: 250,000, 750,000, 1,500,000 units in vials for reconstitution

Indications & dosages
➤ *Atrioventous cannula occlusion*—**Adult:** 250,000 units in 2 ml IV solution in each cannula limb over 25-35 min. Clamp cannula × 2 hr. Aspirate, flush, and reconnect.
➤ *Venous thrombosis, PE, arterial thrombosis and embolism*—**Adult:** 250,000 units IV over 30 min. Then 100,000 units/hr IV × 72 hr for DVT and 100,000 units/

---

§ Adjust in immunocompromised patients   ¶ Adjust in debilitated patients

hr × 24-72 hr for PE and arterial thrombosis or embolism.

➤ *Lysis of coronary artery thrombi*—**Adult:** 20,000 units bolus via coronary catheter; then 2,000 units/min infusion over 60 min. Or, as IV infusion. Usual adult dose 1.5 million units IV over 60 min.

sucralfate
Carafate, Sulcrate*

Pepsin inhibitor; antiulcer drug
PRC: B

Available forms
Suspension: 1 g/10 ml; *Tablets:* 1 g

Indications & dosages
➤ *Duodenal ulcer (≤ 8 wk)*—**Adult:** 1 g PO qid 1 hr pc and hs.
➤ *Maintenance treatment of duodenal ulcer*—**Adult:** 1 g PO bid.

sulfasalazine (salazosulfapyridine, sulphasalazine)
Azulfidine, Azulfidine EN-tabs

Sulfonamide; antibiotic
PRC: B

Available forms
Tablets: 500 mg; *Tablets (delayed-release):* 500 mg

Indications & dosages
➤ *Ulcerative colitis, Crohn's disease*—**Adult:** 3-4 g/d PO in evenly divided doses; maintenance 2 g/d PO in divided doses q 6 hr. **Child > 2 yr:** 40-60 mg/kg/d PO, divided into 3-6 doses; then 30 mg/kg/d in 4 doses.
➤ *RA*—**Adult:** 2-3 g/d in 2 divided doses.
➤ *Juvenile RA*—**Child ≥ 6 yr:** 30-50 mg/kg (delayed-release tablet) PO daily in 2 divided doses. Max 2 g/d. To reduce GI upset, start with ¼-⅓ of maintenance dose and increase q wk × 1 mo.

sulindac
Apo-Sulin*, Clinoril, Novo-Sundac*

NSAID; nonopioid analgesic, anti-inflammatory
PRC: NR

Available forms
Tablets: 150, 200 mg

Indications & dosages
➤ *OA, RA, ankylosing spondylitis*—**Adult:** 150 mg PO bid; increase to 200 mg bid prn.
➤ *Subacromial bursitis, supraspinatus tendinitis, gouty arthritis*—**Adult:** 200 mg PO bid × 7-14 d. Reduce as symptoms subside.

sumatriptan succinate
Imitrex, Imitrex Nasal Spray

Selective 5-hydroxytryptamine receptor agonist; antimigraine drug
PRC: C

Available forms
Injection: 6 mg/0.5 ml in 0.5-ml prefilled syringes, vials; *Spray:* 5, 20 mg/0.1 ml; *Tablets:* 25, 50, 100 mg (base)

Indications & dosages

➤ *Migraine*—**Adult:** 6 mg SC. Max two 6-mg injections daily ≥ 1 hr apart. Or, initial dose 25-100 mg PO; 2nd dose ≤ 100 mg in 2 hr prn. Then, more doses q 2 hr prn; max PO dose 200 mg/d. Or, 5, 10, or 20 mg intranasally into 1 nostril. May repeat once after 2 hr; max 40 mg/d.‡

tacrine hydrochloride
Cognex

Cholinesterase inhibitor; psycho-therapeutic
PRC: C

Available forms
Capsules: 10, 20, 30, 40 mg

Indications & dosages
➤ *Alzheimer's dementia*—**Adult:** 10 mg PO qid. After 6 wk (if tolerated with no increase in transaminase), 20 mg qid. After 6 wk, 30 mg qid. If still tolerated, 40 mg qid after another 6 wk.

tacrolimus
Protopic

Macrolide; immunosuppressant
PRC: C

Available forms
Ointment: 0.03, 0.1%

Indications & dosages
➤ *Moderate-to-severe atopic dermatitis where other treatment is inadequate or contraindicated*—**Adult:** Thin layer of 0.03% or 0.1% ointment to affected area

bid × 1 wk after area clears. **Child ≥ 2 yr:** Thin layer of 0.03% ointment to affected area bid × 1 wk after area clears.

tamoxifen citrate
Nolvadex, Nolvadex-D*

Nonsteroidal antiestrogen; antineoplastic
PRC: D

Available forms
Tablets: 10, 20 mg; *Tablets (enteric-coated)**: 10, 20 mg

Indications & dosages
➤ *Breast CA*—**Adult:** 20-40 mg PO daily. Give doses > 20 mg in 2 divided doses.
➤ *Ductal carcinoma in situ; reduce risk of invasive breast CA after breast surgery and radiation; reduce risk of breast CA in high-risk women*—**Adult:** 20 mg PO daily × 5 yr.

tamsulosin hydrochloride
Flomax

Alpha$_{1a}$-antagonist; BPH drug
PRC: B

Available forms
Capsule: 0.4 mg

Indications & dosages
➤ *BPH*—**Adult:** 0.4 mg PO daily. If no response after 2-4 wk, increase to 0.8 mg PO daily. If treatment interrupted × several d, restart at 1 capsule daily.

§ Adjust in immunocompromised patients   ¶ Adjust in debilitated patients

tegaserod maleate
Zelnorm

5-HT₄ receptor partial agonist; irritable bowel agent
PRC: B

Available forms
Tablets: 2, 6 mg

Indications & dosages
➤ *IBS with constipation*—**Women:** 6 mg PO bid ac × 4-6 wk. May repeat × 4-6 wk.

temazepam
Restoril

Benzodiazepine; sedative-hypnotic
PRC: X; CSS: IV

Available forms
Capsules: 15, 30 mg

Indications & dosages
➤ *Insomnia*—**Adult:** 7.5-30 mg PO hs.¶
Elderly: 7.5 mg PO hs.

tenecteplase
TNKase

Recombinant tissue plasminogen activator; thrombolytic
PRC: C

Available forms
Injection: 50 mg

Indications & dosages
➤ *MI*—**Adult < 60 kg:** 30 mg IV over 5 sec. **Adult 60-69 kg:** 35 mg IV over 5 sec. **Adult 70-79 kg:** 40 mg IV over 5 sec. **Adult 80-89 kg:** 45 mg IV over 5 sec. **Adult ≥ 90 kg:** 50 mg IV over 5 sec. Max 50 mg.

tenofovir disoproxil fumarate
Viread

Nucleotide reverse transcriptase inhibitor; antiviral, antiretroviral
PRC: B

Available forms
Tablets: 300 mg as the fumarate salt (equivalent to 245 mg of tenofovir disoproxil)

Indications & dosages
➤ *HIV-1 infection, with other antiretroviral drugs*—**Adult:** 300 mg PO daily with meal. Give 2 hr before or 1 hr after didanosine.

terazosin hydrochloride
Hytrin

Selective alpha₁ blocker; antihypertensive
PRC: C

Available forms
Tablets, capsules: 1, 2, 5, 10 mg

Indications & dosages
➤ *HTN*—**Adult:** 1 mg PO hs. Adjust prn. Range 1-5 mg/d; max 20 mg/d.
➤ *Symptomatic BPH*—**Adult:** 1 mg PO hs. Increase stepwise to 2, 5, or 10 mg/d; usually 10 mg/d.

terbinafine hydrochloride (oral)
Lamisil

Synthetic allylamine derivative; antifungal
PRC: B

Available forms
Tablets: 250 mg

Indications & dosages
➤ *Tinea unguium*—**Adult:** 250 mg PO daily × 6 wk (fingernail) or × 12 wk (toenail).

terbutaline sulfate
Brethine, Bricanyl

Beta$_2$ adrenergic agonist; bronchodilator, premature labor inhibitor (tocolytic)
PRC: B

Available forms
Injection: 1 mg/ml; *Tablets:* 2.5, 5 mg

Indications & dosages
➤ *Bronchospasm*—**Adult, child ≥ 12 yr:** 0.25 mg SC; repeat in 15-30 min prn. Max 0.5 mg in 4 hr. Or, 2.5-5 mg PO q 6 hr tid. Max 15 mg/d. **Child 12-15 yr:** 2.5 mg PO q 6 hr tid while awake. Max 7.5 mg/d.

teriparatide
Forteo

Biosynthetic parathyroid hormone; antiosteoporotic
PRC: C

Available forms
Injection: 250 mcg/ml

Indications & dosages
➤ *Osteoporosis in high-risk postmenopausal women and in high-risk men*—**Adult:** 20 mcg SC daily.

testosterone
Testamone 100

testosterone cypionate
Depo-Testosterone

testosterone propionate
Testex

testosterone transdermal system
Androderm, Testoderm

Androgen; androgen replacement, antineoplastic
PRC: X; CSS: III

Available forms
testosterone *Injection (aqueous suspension):* 25, 50, 100 mg/ml; **cypionate** *Injection (in oil):* 100, 200 mg/ml; **propionate** *Injection (in oil):* 50, 100 mg/ml; **transdermal system** *Transdermal patch:* 2.5, 4, 5, 6 mg/d

Indications & dosages
➤ *Hypogonadism*—**Adult (man):** testosterone propionate 10-25 mg IM 2-3 times/wk; or **testosterone cypionate** 50-400 mg IM q 2-4 wk.
➤ *Breast CA 1-5 yr postmenopausal*—**Adult (woman):** 100 mg IM 2 times/wk; **testosterone propionate** 50-100 mg IM 3 times/wk; or **testosterone cypionate** 200-400 mg IM q 2-4 wk.

---

§ Adjust in immunocompromised patients ¶ Adjust in debilitated patients

➤ *Primary, hypogonadotropic hypogonadism*—**Adult (man): Testoderm** One 4-6 mg/d patch on scrotal area daily. Patch worn × 22-24 hr/d; or, **Androderm** Two systems applied pm. Apply to clean, dry skin on back, abdomen, upper arms, or thigh.

---

tetracycline hydrochloride
Achromycin, Apo-Tetra*, Novo-Tetra*, Nu-Tetra*, Sumycin, Topicycline*

Tetracycline; antibiotic
PRC: D

Available forms
Capsules: 250, 500 mg; *Ointment:* 3%; *Oral suspension:* 125 mg/5 ml; *Topical solution:* 2.2 mg/ml

Indications & dosages
➤ *Infection*—**Adult:** 250-500 mg PO q 6 hr. **Child > 8 yr:** 25-50 mg/kg/d PO in divided doses q 6 hr.
➤ *Chlamydia. trachomatis infection*—**Adult:** 500 mg PO qid × 7-21 d.
➤ *Brucellosis*—**Adult:** 500 mg PO q 6 hr × 3 wk with streptomycin IM.

---

theophylline
Immediate-release: Bronkodyl, Slo-Phyllin; timed-release: Aerolate, Theochron, Theolair, Theo-Sav, T-Phyl, Uniphyl

theophylline sodium glycinate

Xanthine derivative; bronchodilator
PRC: C

Available forms
Capsules: 100, 200 mg; *Capsules (extended-release):* 50, 60, 65, 75, 100, 125, 130, 200, 250, 260, 300 mg; *D₅W Injection:* 200 mg in 50, 100 ml; 400 mg in 100, 250, 500, 1,000 ml; 800 mg in 250, 500, 1,000 ml; *Elixir, oral solution, syrup:* 27, 50 mg/5 ml; *Tablets:* 100, 125, 200, 250, 300 mg; *Tablets (chewable):* 100 mg; *Tablets (extended-release):* 100, 200, 250, 300, 400, 500, 600 mg

Indications & dosages
➤ *Acute bronchospasm if not using drug*—IV loading dose 4.7 mg/kg slowly; then maintenance. **Adult (nonsmoker):** 6 mg/kg PO; then 2-3 mg/kg q 6 hr × 2 doses. Maintenance 3 mg/kg q 8 hr. Or, 0.55 mg/kg/hr IV × 12 hr; then 0.39 mg/kg/hr. **Adult (healthy smoker) and child 9-16 yr:** 6 mg/kg PO; then 3 mg/kg q 4 hr × 3 doses. Maintenance 3 mg/kg q 6 hr. Or, 0.79 mg/kg/hr IV × 12 hr; then 0.63 mg/kg/hr. **Adult with HF, liver disease:** 6 mg/kg PO; then 2 mg/kg q 8 hr × 2 doses. Maintenance 1-2 mg/kg q 12 hr. Or, 0.39 mg/kg/hr IV × 12 hr; then 0.08-0.16 mg/kg/hr. **Child 6 mo-9 yr:** 6 mg/kg PO; then 4 mg/kg q 4 hr × 3 doses. Maintenance 4 mg/kg q 6 hr. Or, 0.95 mg/kg/hr IV × 12 hr; then 0.79 mg/kg/hr.
➤ *Chronic bronchospasm*—**Adult, child:** 16 mg/kg or 400 mg PO daily in 3-4 divided doses q 6-8 hr; or 12 mg/kg or 400 mg PO daily (extended-release) in 2-3 divided doses q 8 or 12 hr. Increase as tolerated q 2-3 d to max. **Child > 16 yr:** 13 mg/kg or

---

900 mg PO daily in divided doses. **Child 12-16 yr:** 18 mg/kg PO daily in divided doses. **Child 9-12 yr:** 20 mg/kg PO daily in divided doses. **Child < 9 yr:** 24 mg/kg/d PO in divided doses.

thiamine hydrochloride (vitamin B₁)
Biamine

Water-soluble vitamin; nutritional supplement
PRC: A

Available forms
Elixir*: 250 mcg/5 ml; *Injection:* 100 mg/ml; *Tablets:* 25, 50, 100, 250, 500 mg; *Tablets (enteric-coated):* 20 mg

Indications & dosages
➤ *Beriberi*—**Adult:** 10-20 mg IM tid × 2 wk; then diet correction and multivitamin containing 5-10 mg/d thiamine × 1 mo. **Child:** 10-50 mg/d IM × several wk with adequate diet.
➤ *Wernicke's encephalopathy*—**Adult:** 100 mg IV; then 50-100 mg/d IV or IM until patient eats balanced diet.

thioridazine hydrochloride
Apo-Thioridazine*, Mellaril, Mellaril Concentrate, Novo-Ridazine*, PMS Thioridazine*

Phenothiazine (piperidine derivative); antipsychotic
PRC: NR

Available forms
Oral concentrate: 30, 100 mg/ml (3-4.2% alcohol); *Oral suspension:* 25, 100 mg/5 ml; *Tablets:* 10, 15, 25, 50, 100, 150, 200 mg

Indications & dosages
➤ *Psychosis*—**Adult:** 50-100 mg PO tid; slowly increase to 800 mg/d in divided doses prn.
➤ *Depression with anxiety (short-term), multiple symptoms in elderly*—**Adult:** 25 mg PO tid. Maintenance 20-200 mg/d. Max 200 mg/d. **Child 2-12 yr:** 0.5-3 mg/kg PO daily in divided doses.

thiothixene
Navane

thiothixene hydrochloride
Navane

Thioxanthene; antipsychotic
PRC: NR

Available forms
thiothixene *Capsules:* 1, 2, 5, 10, 20 mg; **hydrochloride** *Injection:* 2, 5 mg/ml; *Oral concentrate:* 5 mg/ml (7% alcohol)

Indications & dosages
➤ *Psychosis*—**Adult:** 2 mg PO tid. Increase to 15 mg/d.
➤ *Severe psychosis*—**Adult:** 5 mg PO bid. Increase to 20-30 mg/d. Max 60 mg/d. Or, 4 mg IM bid or qid. Max 30 mg/d IM. Replace with PO ASAP.

---

§ Adjust in immunocompromised patients ¶ Adjust in debilitated patients

ticarcillin disodium
Ticar

Extended-spectrum PCN, alpha-carboxypenicillin; antibiotic
PRC: B

Available forms
Powder for injection: 1, 3, 6 g; *IV infusion:* 3 g

Indications & dosages
➤ *Serious infection*—**Adult:** 200-300 mg/kg IV daily in divided doses q 4-6 hr.†,‡ **Child < 40 kg:** 200-300 mg/kg IV daily in divided doses q 4-6 hr.†, ‡ **Neonate > 2 kg:** 225-300 mg/kg daily in divided doses q 8 hr IM or IV over 10-20 min.†,‡ **Neonate < 2 kg:** 150-225 mg/kg daily in divided doses q 8-12 hr IM or IV over 10-20 min.†, ‡
➤ *UTI*—**Adult, child:** Complicated infection, 150-200 mg/kg IV daily in divided doses q 4-6 hr. **Adult:** Uncomplicated infection, 1 g IV or IM q 6 hr.†, ‡ **Child < 40 kg:** Uncomplicated infection, 50-100 mg/kg daily IM or direct IV divided q 6-8 hr.†, ‡

ticarcillin disodium and clavulanate potassium
Timentin

Beta-lactamase inhibitor; antibiotic
PRC: B

Available forms
Injection: 3 g ticarcillin and 100 mg clavulanic acid

Indications & dosages
➤ *UTI; lower respiratory tract, bone and joint, skin and skin-structure infection; septicemia*—**Adult:** 3.1 g IV infusion q 4-6 hr.†

ticlopidine hydrochloride
Ticlid

Platelet aggregation inhibitor; antithrombotic
PRC: B

Available forms
Tablets: 250 mg

Indications & dosages
➤ *Reduce risk of thrombotic stroke*—**Adult:** 250 mg PO bid with meals.

timolol maleate (ophthalmic)
Betimol, Timoptic, Timoptic-XE

Beta blocker; antiglaucoma agent
PRC: C

Available forms
Ophthalmic solution, gel: 0.25, 0.5%

Indications & dosages
➤ *Chronic glaucoma, elevated IOP from ocular HTN*—**Adult:** 1 gtt 0.25% solution in each affected eye bid; maintenance 1 gtt/d. If no response, 1 gtt 0.5% solution bid. If IOP is controlled, reduce to 1 gtt/d. Or, 1 gtt gel daily.

---

timolol maleate (systemic)
Apo-Timol*, Blocadren

Beta blocker; antihypertensive, adjunct in MI treatment
PRC: C

Available forms
Tablets: 5, 10, 20 mg

Indications & dosages
➤ *HTN*—**Adult:** 10 mg PO bid. Max 60 mg/d. Increase q wk prn.
➤ *MI*—**Adult:** 10 mg PO bid.
➤ *Migraine prophylaxis*—**Adult:** 20 mg PO daily in 1 or divided doses bid. Increase prn to max 30 mg/d.

tinzaparin sodium
Innohep

Low–molecular-weight heparin; anticoagulant
PRC: B

Available forms
Injection: 20,000 anti-Xa IU per ml in 2-ml vials

Indications & dosages
➤ *Symptomatic DVT with or without PE*—**Adult:** 175 anti-Xa IU/kg of body wt SC daily × ≥ 6 d and until patient is adequately anticoagulated with warfarin (INR ≥ 2.0) × 2 consecutive d. Warfarin treatment should begin when appropriate, usually within 1-3 d after tinzaparin starts. Volume to be given may be calculated as follows: Patient wt in kg × 0.00875 ml/kg = volume to be given (in ml)

tobramycin
AKTob, Tobrex

Aminoglycoside; antibiotic
PRC: B

Available forms
Ophthalmic ointment, solution: 0.3%

Indications & dosages
➤ *Ocular infection*—**Adult, child:** 1-2 gtt into affected eye q 4 hr, or thin strip (1 cm) ointment q 8-12 hr. In severe infection, 2 gtt into infected eye q 30-60 min until improvement; then reduce frequency. Or, thin strip ointment q 3-4 hr until improvement; then reduce frequency.

tobramycin sulfate
Nebcin, TOBI

Aminoglycoside; antibiotic
PRC: D

Available forms
Injection: 80, 20 (pediatric) mg/2 ml; *Nebulizer solution (for inhalation):* 300 mg/5 ml; *Powder for injection:* 1.2 g; *Premixed parenteral injection for IV infusion:* 60, 80 mg in NSS

Indications & dosages
➤ *Serious infection*—**Adult:** 3 mg/kg/d IM or IV divided q 8 hr. Max 5 mg/kg/d divided q 6-8 hr for life-threatening infection; reduce to 3 mg/kg/d as soon as indicated. **Child:** 6-7.5 mg/kg/d IM or IV in 3 or 4 equally divided doses. **Neonate < 1 wk, premature infant:** up to 4 mg/kg/d IV or IM in 2 equal doses q 12 hr.†

➤ Pseudomonas aeruginosa *infection in cystic fibrosis*—**Adult, child ≥ 6 yr:** 300 mg q 12 hr via nebulizer × 28 d, followed by 28 d without drug. Repeat cycle.

tolcapone
Tasmar

Catechol-O-methyltransferase inhibitor; antiparkinsonian
PRC: C

Available forms
Tablets: 100, 200 mg

Indications & dosages
➤ *Parkinson's disease*—**Adult:** 100 mg PO tid (with levodopa-carbidopa). Recommended daily dose 100 mg PO tid; 200 mg PO tid can be given, if needed. If giving 200 mg tid and dyskinesia occurs, consider levodopa dose reduction. Max 600 mg/d.†

tolterodine tartrate
Detrol, Detrol LA

Muscarinic receptor antagonist; anticholinergic
PRC: C

Available forms
Capsules (extended-release): 2, 4 mg; *Tablets:* 1, 2 mg

Indications & dosages
➤ *Overactive bladder*—**Adult:** 2 mg PO bid. May lower to 1 mg bid, based on response and tolerance. Or, 4 mg (extended-

release) PO daily. May reduce to 2 mg PO daily (extended-release).‡

topiramate
Topamax

Sulfamate-substituted monosaccharide; antiepileptic
PRC: C

Available forms
Sprinkle capsules: 15, 25 mg; *Tablets:* 25, 100, 200 mg

Indications & dosages
➤ *Partial onset seizures; primary generalized tonic-clonic seizures*—**Adult:** Initiate doses at 25-50 mg/d followed by adjustment of 25-50 mg/wk. Adjust to max 400 mg daily in 2 divided doses.†
➤ *Partial seizures, primary generalized tonic-clonic seizures, or Lennox-Gestaut syndrome*—**Child 2-16 yr:** 5-9 mg/kg/d PO in 2 divided doses. Begin dosage adjustment at 1-3 mg/kg pm × 1 wk. Increase at 1-2 wk intervals by 1-3 mg/kg/d to achieve optimal clinical response. Dosage adjustment should be guided by clinical outcome.†

tramadol hydrochloride
Ultram

Synthetic analgesic; analgesic
PRC: C

Available forms
Tablets: 50 mg

Indications & dosages

➤ *Pain*—**Adult < 75 yr:** 50-100 mg PO q 4-6 hr prn. Max 400 mg/d. **Elderly > 75 yr:** max 300 mg/d in divided doses.†,‡

trazodone hydrochloride
Desyrel

Triazolopyridine derivative; antidepressant
PRC: C

Available forms
Tablets: 50, 100, 150, 300 mg

Indications & dosages

➤ *Depression*—**Adult:** 150 mg PO daily in divided doses; increase by 50 mg/d q 3-4 d prn. Average dose 150-400 mg/d. Max dose 600 mg/d (inpatient); 400 mg/d (outpatient).

treprostinil sodium
Remodulin

Vasodilator; antihypertensive
PRC: B

Available forms
Injection: 1 mg/ml, 2.5 mg/ml, 5 mg/ml, 10 mg/ml

Indications & dosages

➤ *New York Heart Association class II to IV pulmonary arterial hypertension to reduce symptoms caused by exercise*—**Adult:** 1.25 ng/kg/min continuous SC infusion. May reduce to 0.625 ng/kg/min prn. Increase by 1.25-ng/kg/min increments q wk for the 1st 4 wk and then by

≤ 2.5 ng/kg/min each wk for remaining duration of treatment. Max 40 ng/kg/min.‡

tretinoin (retinoic acid, vitamin A acid)
Avita, Renova, Retin-A, Retin-A Micro, Stieva-A*, Stieva-A Forte*

Retinoid, vitamin A derivative; anti-acne agent, anti-wrinkle agent
PRC: C

Available forms
Cream: 0.02, 0.025, 0.05, 0.1%; *Gel:* 0.01, 0.025%; *Microsphere gel:* 0.04%, 0.1%; *Solution:* 0.05%

Indications & dosages

➤ *Acne*—**Adult, child:** Clean affected area and lightly apply daily hs.
➤ *Fine facial wrinkles*—**Adult:** Apply small, pearl-sized amount 0.02% cream to cover area lightly, q pm. May increase to 0.05% cream if skin care, sun avoidance program alone don't work.

triamcinolone acetonide (nasal)
Nasacort, Nasacort AQ

Glucocorticoid; anti-inflammatory
PRC: C

Available forms
Nasal aerosol: 55 mcg/metered spray; *Nasal spray pump:* 55 mcg/spray

Indications & dosages

➤ *Seasonal and perennial allergic rhinitis symptoms*—**Adult, child ≥ 12 yr:**

---

§ Adjust in immunocompromised patients   ¶ Adjust in debilitated patients

Nasacort 2 sprays each nostril daily; max 4 sprays per nostril daily prn. Or, **Nasacort AQ** 2 sprays each nostril daily; decrease to 1 spray each nostril daily for allergic disorders. **Child 6-12 yr: Nasacort** 2 sprays each nostril daily. Or, **Nasacort AQ** 1 spray each nostril daily. Max 2 sprays each nostril daily.

triamcinolone acetonide (systemic)
Azmacort, Kenalog-10, Triamonide 40, Trilog

Glucocorticoid; anti-inflammatory, anti-asthmatic
PRC: C

Available forms
Inhalation aerosol: 100 mcg/metered spray; *Injection (suspension):* 3, 10, 40 mg/ml; *Tablets:* 1, 2, 4, 8 mg

Indications & dosages
➤ *Inflammation, immunosuppression*—**Adult:** 4-48 mg/d PO in divided doses; 40 mg IM wkly; 1 mg into lesions; 2.5-40 mg into joints or soft tissue.
➤ *Asthma*—**Adult: Azmacort** 2 inhalations tid or qid, or 4 inhalations given bid. Max 16 inhalations/d. **Child 6-12 yr: Azmacort** 1 or 2 inhalations tid or qid, or 2-4 inhalations given bid. Max 12 inhalations/d.

triamcinolone acetonide (topical)
Aristocort, Flutex, Kenalog, Triacet

Topical adrenocorticoid; anti-inflammatory
PRC: C

Available forms
Aerosol: 0.2 mg/2-sec spray; *Cream:* 0.025, 0.1, 0.5%; *Lotion:* 0.025, 0.1%; *Ointment:* 0.025, 0.1, 0.5%; *Paste, solution:* 0.1%

Indications & dosages
➤ *Dermatitis*—**Adult, child:** Apply sparingly bid-qid.
➤ *Inflammation with oral lesions*—**Adult, child:** Apply paste hs and bid or tid prn, preferably pc.

trifluoperazine hydrochloride
Apo-Trifluoperazine*, Solazine*, Stelazine, Terfluzine*

Phenothiazine (piperazine derivative); antipsychotic
PRC: NR

Available forms
Injection: 2 mg/ml; *Oral concentration:* 10 mg/ml; *Tablets:* 1, 2, 5, 10 mg

Indications & dosages
➤ *Anxiety*—**Adult:** 1-2 mg PO bid. Max 6 mg/d. Don't give > 12 wk.
➤ *Schizophrenia, other psychotic disorders*—**Adult:** 2-5 mg PO bid, increase until response. Or, 1-2 mg deep IM q 4-6 hr

---

prn; > 6 mg IM/24 hr rarely needed. **Child 6-12 yr (hospitalized, closely supervised):** 1 mg PO daily or bid; may increase to 15 mg/d.

trihexyphenidyl hydrochloride
Apo-Trihex*, Artane, Trihexane

Anticholinergic; antiparkinsonian
PRC: NR

Available forms
Capsules (sustained-release): 5 mg; *Elixir:* 2 mg/5 ml; *Tablets:* 2, 5 mg

Indications & dosages
➤ *Parkinsonism*—**Adult:** 1 mg PO d 1, 2 mg d 2; then increase by 2 mg q 3-5 d until total of 6-10 mg/d. Give tid with meals or qid or as extended-release form bid. In postencephalitic parkinsonism, 12-15 mg/d may be needed.

triptorelin pamoate
Trelstar Depot, Trelstar LA

Synthetic luteinizing hormone-releasing hormone (LHRH) analogue; antineoplastic
PRC: X

Available forms
Injection: 3.75-, 11.25-mg single-dose vials and Debioclip single-dose delivery system

Indications & dosages
➤ *Palliative treatment of advanced prostate CA*—**Adult:** 3.75 mg IM (Trelstar Depot) q mo as single injection or 11.25 mg IM (Trelstar LA) given q 84 d as single injection.

valacyclovir hydrochloride
Valtrex

Synthetic purine nucleoside; antiviral
PRC: B

Available forms
Caplets: 500, 1,000 mg

Indications & dosages
➤ *Herpes zoster (shingles)*—**Adult:** 1 g PO tid × 7 d.†
➤ *Initial genital herpes*—**Adult:** 1 g PO bid × 10 d.†
➤ *Recurrent genital herpes*—**Adult:** 500 mg PO bid × 3 d at 1st sign.†,§
➤ *Chronic suppressive treatment of recurrent genital herpes*—**Adult:** 1 g PO daily. Patient with ≤ 9 episodes/yr can take 500 mg PO daily.†,§
➤ *Cold sores (herpes labialis)*—**Adult:** 2 g PO × 2 doses, about 12 hr apart.†

valdecoxib
Bextra

COX-2 inhibitor; NSAID
PRC: C

Available forms
Tablets: 10, 20 mg

Indications & dosages
➤ *OA, RA*—**Adult:** 10 mg PO daily.
➤ *Primary dysmenorrhea*—**Adult:** 20 mg PO bid prn.

§ Adjust in immunocompromised patients ¶ Adjust in debilitated patients

valganciclovir
Valcyte

Synthetic nucleoside; antiviral
PRC: C

Available forms
Tablets: 450 mg

Indications & dosages
➤ *Active CMV retinitis in AIDS*—**Adult:** 900 mg PO bid with food × 21 d. Maintenance dose 900 mg PO daily with food.†
➤ *Inactive CMV retinitis*—**Adult:** 900 mg PO daily with food.†

valproate sodium
Depacon, Depakene Syrup

valproic acid
Depakene

divalproex sodium
Depakote, Depakote ER, Depakote Sprinkle, Epival*

Carboxylic acid derivative; anticonvulsant
PRC: D

Available forms
valproate *Injection:* 100 mg/ml; *Syrup:* 250 mg/5 ml; **valproic** *Capsules:* 250 mg; **divalproex** *Capsules (sprinkle):* 125 mg; *Tablets (delayed-release):* 125, 250, 500 mg; *Tablets (extended-release):* 500 mg

Indications & dosages
➤ *Simple and complex absence seizures, mixed seizure types (including absence seizures)*—**Adult, child:** 15 mg/kg PO or IV daily; increase by 5-10 mg/kg/d q wk to max 60 mg/kg/d.
➤ *Mania*—**Adult:** divalproex sodium 750 mg/d in divided doses. Adjust prn; max 60 mg/kg/d.
➤ *Migraine prophylaxis*—**Adult: divalproex sodium** 250 mg (delayed-release) PO bid; increase to 1,000 mg/d prn. Or, **Depakote ER** 500 mg PO daily × 1 wk, then 1,000 mg PO daily.
➤ *Complex partial seizures*—**Adult, child ≥ 10 yr:** 10-15 mg/kg PO or IV daily; increase by 5-10 mg/kg/d q wk to max 60 mg/kg/d.
Elderly: Start at lower dose and adjust dose more slowly. Regularly monitor fluid and nutritional intake, dehydration, somnolence, and other adverse events.

valsartan
Diovan

Angiotensin II antagonist; antihypertensive
PRC: C (D, 2nd and 3rd trimesters)

Available forms
Tablets: 80, 160, 320 mg

Indications & dosages
➤ *HTN*—**Adult:** 80 mg PO daily. BP reduction in 2-4 wk. For greater effect, increase to 160 or 320 mg/d or add diuretic.
➤ *HF (New York Heart Association class II-IV) in patients intolerant of ACE inhibitors*—**Adult:** 40 mg PO bid. Increase as tolerated to 80 mg bid. Max dose 160 mg bid. Consider reduction in diuretic use.

---

*Canadian   † Adjust in renal impairment   ‡ Adjust in liver impairment

Use with an ACE inhibitor and a beta blocker is not recommended.

vancomycin hydrochloride
Lyphocin, Vancocin, Vancoled

Glycopeptide; antibiotic
PRC: C

Available forms
Capsules: 125, 250 mg; *IV infusion (frozen):* 500 mg/100 ml D₅W; *Powder for injection:* 500-mg, 1-g vial; *Powder for oral solution:* 1-, 10-g bottle

Indications & dosages
➤ *Serious infection*—**Adult:** 1-1.5 g IV q 12 hr. **Child:** 10 mg/kg IV q 6 hr. **Neonate, young infant:** 15 mg/kg IV; then 10 mg/kg IV q 12 hr if < 1 wk of age, and 10 mg/kg IV q 8 hr if > 1 wk of age but < 1 mo of age.†
➤ *Pseudomembranous and staphylococcal enterocolitis from antibiotics*—**Adult:** 125-500 mg PO q 6 h × 7-10 d. **Child:** 40 mg/kg PO daily in divided doses q 6 hr × 7-10 d. Max 2 g/d.†
➤ *Endocarditis prophylaxis (dental procedures)*—**Adult, child > 27 kg:** 1 g IV over 1 hr starting 1 hr before procedure. **Child < 27 kg:** 20 mg/kg IV over 1-2 hr; ending within 30 min of start of procedure.†

venlafaxine hydrochloride
Effexor, Effexor XR

SSRI, norepinephrine, dopamine reuptake inhibitor; antidepressant
PRC: C

Available forms
Capsules (extended-release): 37.5, 75, 150 mg; *Tablets:* 25, 37.5, 50, 75, 100 mg

Indications & dosages
➤ *Depression, anxiety*—**Adult:** 75 mg PO daily in 2 or 3 divided doses with food. For anxiety, use extended-release. Increase prn by 75 mg/d at intervals ≥ 4 d. Moderate depression, max 225 mg/d; severe depression, max 375 mg/d.

verapamil hydrochloride
Apo-Verap*, Calan, Calan SR, Covera-HS, Isoptin SR, Novo-Veramil*, Nu-Verap*, Verelan, Verelan PM

Calcium channel blocker; antianginal, antihypertensive, antiarrhythmic
PRC: C

Available forms
Capsules (extended-release): 120, 180, 240 mg; *Capsules (sustained-release):* 120, 160*, 180, 240, 360 mg; *Injection:* 2.5 mg/ml; *Tablets:* 40, 80, 120 mg; *Tablets (extended-release):* 100, 120, 180, 200, 240, 300 mg; *Tablets (sustained-release):* 120, 180, 240 mg

Indications & dosages
➤ *Vasospastic angina, chronic angina, chronic atrial fibrillation*—**Adult:** 80-120 mg PO tid. Increase q wk prn. Max 480 mg/d.
➤ *Supraventricular arrhythmias*—**Adult:** 0.075-0.15 mg/kg IV push over 2 min; 0.15 mg/kg in 30 min prn. **Child < 1 yr:** 0.1-0.2 mg/kg IV over 2 min. **Child 1-**

15 yr: 0.1-0.3 mg/kg IV over 2 min. For child, may repeat in 30 min.
➤ *HTN*—**Adult:** 120-240 mg PO daily of extended-release capsules or tablets in am; may increase by 120 mg increments. Or, **Covera-HS** 180 mg PO hs of extended-release core tablets; may increase to 240 mg PO daily; may be further increased by 120 mg increments to max 480 mg. Or, **Verelan-PM** 200 mg PO daily of controlled extended-release capsule; may increase to 300-400 mg PO hs. Or, 40 mg PO bid to 80 mg PO tid of immediate-release preparation; max 360-480 mg PO daily.

vinblastine sulfate (VLB)
Velban, Velbe*

Vinca alkaloid; antineoplastic
PRC: D

Available forms
Injection: 10-mg vial (lyophilized powder), 1 mg/ml in 10-ml vials

Indications & dosages
➤ *Breast, testicular CA; Hodgkin's disease; malignant lymphoma*—**Adult:** 3.7 mg/m² IV q 1-2 wk. Max 18.5 mg/m² IV q wk. Don't repeat if WBC < 4,000/mm³. **Child:** 2.5 mg/m² IV q wk. Increase by 1.25 mg/m² until WBC < 3,000/mm³ or tumor response seen. Max 12.5 mg/m² IV q wk.‡

vincristine sulfate (VCR)
Oncovin, Vincasar PFS

Vinca alkaloid, antineoplastic
PRC: D

Available forms
Injection: 1 mg/ml in 1-, 2-, 5-ml multidose and preservative-free vials

Indications & dosages
➤ *Acute lymphoblastic leukemia, other leukemias; Hodgkin's disease*—**Adult:** 1.4 mg/m² IV q wk. Max 2 mg/wk. **Child > 10 kg:** 2 mg/m² IV q wk. **Child ≤ 10 kg or body surface area < 1 m²:** Initially, 0.05 mg/kg IV q wk.

voriconazole
Vfend

Synthetic triazole; antifungal
PRC: D

Available forms
Injection: 200 mg; *Tablets:* 50, 200 mg

Indications & dosages
➤ *Invasive aspergillosis; serious infections caused by* Fusarium *species and* Scedosporium apiospermum *in patients intolerant of or refractory to other therapy*—**Adult:** 6 mg/kg IV q 12 hr × 2 doses, then 4 mg/kg IV q 12 hr. Switch to PO form as tolerated, using maintenance doses‡: **Adults ≥ 40 kg:** 200 mg PO q 12 hr. May increase to 300 mg PO q 12 hr prn.‡ **Adults < 40 kg:** 100 mg PO q 12 hr. May increase to 150 mg PO q 12 hr prn.‡

---

warfarin sodium
Coumadin, Panwarfin, Sofarin, Warfilone

Coumarin derivative; anticoagulant
PRC: X

Available forms
Powder for injection: 2 mg/ml; *Tablets:* 1, 2, 2.5, 3, 4, 5, 6, 7.5, 10 mg

Indications & dosages
➤ *PE with DVT, MI, rheumatic heart disease with heart valve damage, prosthetic heart valves, chronic atrial fibrillation—* **Adult:** 2-5 mg PO daily × 2-4 d; then dose based on daily PT and INR. Maintenance 2-10 mg PO daily.

zafirlukast
Accolate

Antileukotriene; anti-inflammatory
PRC: B

Available forms
Tablets: 10, 20 mg

Indications & dosages
➤ *Asthma—***Adult, child ≥ 12 yr:** 20 mg PO bid 1 hr ac or 2 hr pc. **Child 5-11 yr:** 10 mg PO bid.

zalcitabine (ddC, dideoxycytidine)
Hivid

Nucleoside analogue; antiviral
PRC: C

Available forms
Tablets: 0.375, 0.75 mg

Indications & dosages
➤ *Advanced HIV infection—***Adult, child ≥ 13 yr:** 0.75 mg PO q 8 hr with zidovudine 200 mg PO q 8 hr.†

zaleplon
Sonata

Pyrazolopyrimidine; hypnotic
PRC: C; CSS: IV

Available forms
Capsules: 5, 10 mg

Indications & dosages
➤ *Insomnia (short-term)—***Adult:** 10 mg PO daily hs; increase to 20 mg prn. Low-wt adult may respond to 5-mg dose.‡,¶

zanamivir
Relenza

Neuraminidase inhibitor; antiviral
PRC: B

Available forms
Powder for inhalation: 5 mg/blister

Indications & dosages
➤ *Symptomatic influenza virus ≤ 2 d—* **Adult, child ≥ 7 yr:** 2 oral inhalations (total dose 10 mg) q 12 hr using Diskhaler × 5 d. Give 2 doses on 1st d if ≥ 2 hr between doses.

---

§ Adjust in immunocompromised patients   ¶ Adjust in debilitated patients

zidovudine (azidothymidine, AZT)
Apo-Zidovudine*, Novo-AZT*, Retrovir

Thymidine analogue; antiviral
PRC: C

Available forms
Capsules: 100 mg; *Injection:* 10 mg/ml; *Syrup:* 50 mg/5 ml; *Tablets:* 300 mg

Indications & dosages
➤ *HIV infection*—**Adult, child ≥ 12 yr:** 600 mg/d PO in divided doses with other antiretroviral agents. Or, 1 mg/kg IV over 1 hr q 4 hr until patient can tolerate oral therapy. **Child 6 wk-12 yr:** 160 mg/m² PO q 8 hr (480 mg/m²/d to max 200 mg q 8 hr) or 120 mg/m² IV q 6 hr by intermittent infusion or 20 mg/m²/hr by continuous infusion with other antiretroviral agents.†,‡
➤ *Prevention of maternal-fetal HIV transmission*—**Pregnant woman (initiate at 14-34 wk gestation):** 100 mg PO 5 times/d until start of labor. Then, 2 mg/kg IV over 1 hr followed by continuous IV infusion of 1 mg/kg/hr until umbilical cord is clamped. **Neonate:** 2 mg/kg PO q 6 hr starting within 6-12 hr after birth and continuing until 6 wk old. Or, give 1.5 mg/kg IV over 30 min q 6 hr.†, ‡
Note: Significant anemia (hemoglobin < 7.5 g/dl or reduction of > 25% of baseline) or significant neutropenia (granulocyte count < 750 cells/mm³ or reduction of > 50% from baseline) may require dose interruption until evidence of marrow recovery is observed.

ziprasidone
Geodon

Atypical antipsychotic; psychotropic
PRC: C

Available forms
Capsules: 20, 40, 60, 80 mg; *Injection:* 20 mg/ml single-dose vials (after reconstitution)

Indications & dosages
➤ *Symptomatic schizophrenia*—**Adult:** 20 mg PO bid with food. Dosage adjustments, if necessary, should occur no sooner than q 2 days, but to allow for lowest possible doses, interval should be several wk for symptom response. Effective dosage range 20-80 mg bid. Max 100 mg bid.
➤ *Rapid control of acute agitation in schizophrenia*—**Adult:** 10-20 mg IM prn; max 40 mg/d. Doses of 10 mg may be administered q 2 hr; doses of 20 mg may be administered q 4 hr.

zoledronic acid
Zometa

Bisphosphonate; antihypercalcemic
PRC: D

Available forms
Injection: 4 mg zoledronic acid, 220 mg mannitol, 24 mg sodium citrate

Indications & dosages
➤ *Hypercalcemia from malignancy*—**Adult:** 4 mg IV over ≥ 15 min. If albumin-

corrected serum calcium level doesn't return to normal, consider retreatment with 4 mg. Allow ≥ 7 d to pass before retreatment to allow a full response to initial dose.†

➤ *Multiple myeloma and bone metastases of solid tumors with standard antineoplastic therapy. Prostate CA should have progressed after treatment with at least one hormonal therapy*—**Adult:** 4 mg IV over 15 min q 3-4 wk.†

zolmitriptan
Zomig, Zomig-ZMT

Selective 5-hydroxytryptamine receptor agonist; antimigraine drug
PRC: C

Available forms
Tablets (immediate-release): 2.5, 5 mg; *Tablets (oral disintegrating):* 2.5, 5 mg

Indications & dosages
➤ *Migraine*—**Adult:** 2.5 mg PO; increase to 5 mg/dose prn. If migraine returns, may give 2nd dose after 2 hr. Max 10 mg/24 hr.‡

zolpidem tartrate
Ambien

Imidazopyridine; hypnotic
PRC: B; CSS: IV

Available forms
Tablets: 5, 10 mg

Indications & dosages
➤ *Insomnia (short-term)*—**Adult:** 10 mg PO q hs. **Elderly:** 5 mg PO q hs. Max 10 mg/d.‡

zonisamide
Zonegran

Sulfonamide; anticonvulsant
PRC: C

Available forms
Capsules: 100 mg

Indications & dosages
➤ *Partial seizures*—**Adult, child > 16 yr:** 100 mg PO daily. Increase 100 mg/d q 2 wk prn; max 400 mg/d. Dose > 100 mg, administer daily or divided bid.†,‡

---

§ Adjust in immunocompromised patients　　　　　¶ Adjust in debilitated patients

Dialyzable drugs

The amount of a drug removed by dialysis differs among patients and depends on several factors, including the patient's condition, the drug's properties, length of dialysis and dialysate used, rate of blood flow or dwell time, and purpose of dialysis. Levels of the following drugs are reduced by dialysis.

acetaminophen (may not influence toxicity)
acyclovir
allopurinol
amikacin
amoxicillin
amoxicillin and clavulanate potassium
ampicillin
ampicillin and sulbactam sodium
aspirin
atenolol
azathioprine
aztreonam
captopril
carbenicillin
cefaclor
cefadroxil
cefazolin
cefepime
cefonicid (by 20%)
cefoperazone
cefotaxime
cefotetan (by 20%)
cefoxitin
cefpodoxime
ceftazidime

ceftibuten
ceftizoxime
cefuroxime
cephalexin
cephalothin
cephradine
chloral hydrate
chloramphenicol (by very small amount)
cimetidine
ciprofloxacin (by 20%)
co-trimoxazole
cyclophosphamide
didanosine
disopyramide
enalapril
erythromycin (by 20%)
ethambutol (by 20%)
famciclovir
fluconazole
flucytosine
fluorouracil
foscarnet
gabapentin
ganciclovir
gentamicin

imipenem and cilastatin

isoniazid

kanamycin

ketoprofen

lisinopril

lithium

loracarbef

mercaptopurine

meropenem

methotrexate

methyldopa

metronidazole

mexiletine

minoxidil

nadolol

nelfinavir

netilmicin

nitrofurantoin

nitroprusside

ofloxacin

penicillin G

pentazocine

perindopril

phenobarbital

piperacillin

piperacillin and tazobactam

primidone

procainamide

pyridoxine

quinidine

ranitidine

sotalol

stavudine

streptomycin

sulbactam

sulfamethoxazole

theophylline

ticarcillin

ticarcillin and clavulanate

tobramycin

tocainide

topiramate

trimethoprim

valacyclovir

Look-alike and sound-alike drug names

Watch out for these drug names that resemble other drug names either in the way they're spelled or the way they sound.

abciximab and infliximab

acetazolamide and acetohexamide

acetylcholine and acetylcysteine

Aciphex and Aricept

albuterol and atenolol or Albutein

alitretinoin and tretinoin

amantadine and rimantadine

Ambien and Amen

Amicar and Amikin

amiloride and amiodarone

amiodarone and amiloride

amoxapine and amoxicillin

anakinra and amikacin

Apresoline and Apresazide

Aquasol A and AquaMEPHYTON

Aricept and Ascriptin

Asacol and Os-Cal

Asendin and aspirin

atenolol and timolol or albuterol

Atrovent and Alupent

Avinza and Invanz

baclofen and Bactroban

BCG intravesical and BCG vaccine

Benadryl and Bentyl or Benylin

bepridil and Prepidil

Bumex and Buprenex

bupropion and buspirone

calcifediol and calcitriol

captopril and Capitrol

carboplatin and cisplatin

Cardizem SR and Cardene SR

Celebrex and Cerebyx or Celexa

chlorpromazine and chlorpropamide

cimetidine and simethicone

Citrucel and Citracal

clonidine and quinidine or clomiphene

clotrimazole and co-trimoxazole

clozapine and clofazimine

corticotropin and cosyntropin

Cozaar and Zocor

cyclosporine and cycloserine

desipramine and disopyramide or imipramine

desmopressin and vasopressin

diazoxide and Dyazide

diclofenac and Duphalac

dicyclomine and doxycycline

Dilantin and Dilaudid

dimenhydrinate and diphenhydramine

dipyridamole and disopyramide

disopyramide and desipramine or dipyridamole

dobutamine and dopamine

dronabinol and droperidol

Epogen and Neupogen

Estratab and Estratest

Eurax and Serax

Femara and FemHRT

fentanyl and alfentanil

Flomax and Fosamax

fluoxetine and fluvoxamine

fluticasone and fluconazole

folic acid and folinic acid

Foradil and Toradol

fosinopril and lisinopril

furosemide and torsemide

glimepiride and glyburide or glipizide

hydromorphone and morphine

imipramine and desipramine

Isordil and Isuprel or Inderal

Lamictal and Lamisil

Lantus and Lente

lorazepam and alprazolam

magnesium and manganese

metaproterenol and metoprolol

methylprednisolone and medroxyprogesterone

methyltestosterone and medroxyprogesterone

metoprolol and metaproterenol

Miltown and Milontin

naloxone and naltrexone

Navane and Nubain or Norvasc

nelfinavir and nevirapine

Nicoderm and Nitro-Dur

nifedipine and nimodipine or nicardipine

nitroglycerine and nitroprusside

norepinephrine and epinephrine

Noroxin and Neurontin

nystatin and Nitrostat

olsalazine and olanzapine

paroxetine and paclitaxel

Paxil and Doxil, paclitaxel, or Taxol

pemoline and Pelamine

pentobarbital and phenobarbital

phenytoin and mephenytoin

pioglitazone and rosiglitazone

Pitocin and Pitressin

Plendil and pindolol

prednisolone and prednisone

ProAmatine and protamine

probenecid and Procanbid

procainamide and probenecid

promethazine and promazine

propranolol and Pravachol

ProSom and Proscar, Prozac, or Psorcon

quinidine and clonidine

ranitidine and rimantadine

Restoril and Vistaril

rifabutin and rifampin or rifapentine

risperidone and reserpine

Ritalin and Rifadin

ritodrine and ranitidine

selegiline and Stelazine

Serzone and Seroquel

Sinequan and saquinavir

Solu-Cortef and Solu-Medrol

somatropin and somatrem or sumatriptan

sotalol and Stadol

streptozocin and streptomycin

sulfadiazine and sulfasalazine

sulfamethoxazole and sulfamethizole

sulfisoxazole and sulfasalazine

sumatriptan and somatropin

Tegretol and Toradol

Tenex and Xanax, Entex, or Ten-K

terbutaline and tolbutamide or terbinafine

thioridazine and Thorazine

Tigan and Ticar

trifluoperazine and triflupromazine

Ultracet and Ultracef

valacyclovir and valganciclovir

Vancenase and Vanceril

vinblastine and vincristine

Xanax and Zantac or Tenex

Zyloprim and ZORprin

Zyprexa and Zyrtec

Index

A